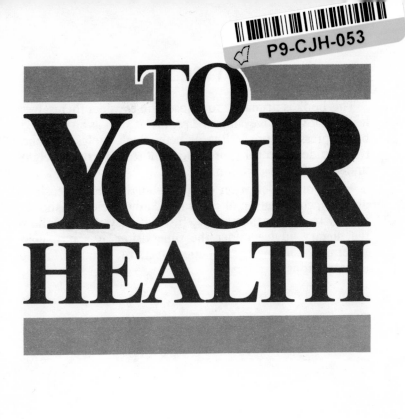

TO YOUR HEALTH

A WORD OF ADVICE_____

This book is primarily for those who consider themselves healthy or who have "minor" problems such as an elevated blood pressure, borderline diabetes, high cholesterol and triglycerides, and for those who want to bring their weight under control in a rational way!

Those on prescription drugs for angina, hypertension, diabetes, claudication or generalized atherosclerosis should not try to doctor themselves. Instead, they should follow the dietary advice under the supervision of a physician experienced in the therapeutic effects of dietary lifestyle modifications.

Library of Congress catalog card number: 87-90391

EDITOR: Jac Flanders
COVER DESIGN: Richard Tinker

Printed in the United States of America

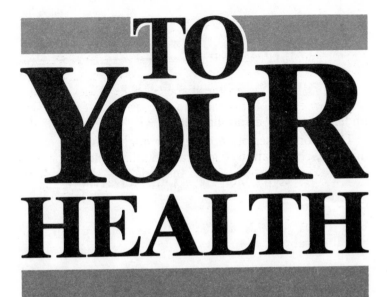

TO YOUR HEALTH

HOW TO EAT MORE AND LIVE LONGER AND BETTER

Dr. HANS DIEHL

Published by
THE QUIET HOUR
630 Brookside Avenue
Redlands, California 92373-4699

ACKNOWLEDGEMENTS_____

My deep appreciation and gratitude go to:

Jac Flanders, for spending countless hours in shaping and editing the manuscript.

Aileen Ludington, M.D., for her work as advisor and medical copy editor. Helen Little, for serving as manuscript editor.

Ellis Jones, for his artistic skills in doing the graphic illustrations.

Ralph Graham, M.D., and the Lassen Foundation for their support of this health enhancement effort.

Lee and Linda Stanley of Morning Star Productions for their perception and shaping of a creative film product.

Sue Davis and Joyce Hack, dietitians, and Shirley Venden. for their contributions in the recipe section.

The Quiet Hour, for their support and Christian commitment and dedication to film, radio and printed production, all designed to contribute to the making of fuller, happier and healthier lives.

The Publishers, for giving permission to reprint excerpts of the following books:
The Pritikin Program for Diet and Exercise by N. Pritikin with P. McGrady. NY: Grosset & Dunlap, 1979. (pp. 159-161)
The Living Heart by M. deBakey, A. Gotto et al. NY: Raven Press, 1984 (p. 96, Fig. 8.4)
The McDougall Plan for Super Health & Life-long Weight Loss by J. and M. McDougall. Piscataway, NJ: New Century Publ., 1983. (P. 19, Fig. 2.3)

DEDICATION————————————

To my wife *Lily* and our children, *Byron* and *Carmen*.

To the memory of *Ellen G. White* and *John Harvey Kellogg,* M.D., great pioneers who more than one hundred years ago laid the foundation for a genuine large-scale health rejuvenation by advocating a simpler diet and lifestyle.

To the memory of *Nathan Pritikin* who enriched my professional life and who made the quantum leap from theory to practice for a sound treatment and prevention approach to America's lifestyle-related killer diseases.

To patients and participants who have attended my programs, lectures and seminars on three continents and who have gone on to validate many of the outlined dietary principles by dramatically improving and enhancing their health and the quality of their lives. Their success motivated me to move ahead, committed to reaching more people and serving them through the communication media.

To all those who are willing to learn how to live with ALL their hearts!

> *Dr. Hans A. Diehl*
> Loma Linda, CA
> January 1987

The first recorded controlled dietary experiment.

" 'Please, give to your servants a ten days' test, allowing us to eat vegetables and to drink water. Then compare our looks with that of the other youths, who have eaten of the king's menu, and act according to your findings.' He agreed with them on this score, gave them a ten days' test, and after ten days they looked healthier and were in better condition than the youths who were eating the royal dishes; so the overseer discontinued their royal rations of meat and wine and served them vegetables."
—Daniel 1:12-16, *The Holy Bible,* The New Berkeley Version

"The doctor of the future will give no medicine, but will interest his patient in the core of the human frame, in diet, and in the cause and prevention of disease."

—Thomas A. Edison

"You can do more for your own health and well-being than any doctor, any hospital, any drugs, any exotic medical device."
—Joseph Califano as Secretary of
Health, Education and Welfare

"Health is not everything. But without it, everything is nothing."

—Hans A. Diehl

TABLE OF CONTENTS————————————

Eat Yourself Healthy!

Having practiced cardiology for more than 20 years and having been carefully trained in rehabilitating victims of cardiovascular disease by means of pharmaceutical and surgical interventions, I have been increasingly impressed during the last 10 years at the effectiveness of the lifestyle medicine approach to these diseases. The potential for returning patients with degenerative diseases to normal function, of reducing or stopping their medications, and often obviating their need for surgery, has been truly astounding.

During these years I have worked with hundreds of patients. Most of these patients, often within weeks, were able to lower their blood pressure levels and get off blood pressure medication. Almost all were able to discontinue their diabetic drugs and insulin injections with blood sugar levels controlled. Many were able to lose weight rationally and successfully and to keep it off without being on semi-starvation diets. And many reduced their blood cholesterol levels substantially and their requirements for angina medication. Basically, what they did was to eat a more natural diet of food-as-grown and get into a regular walking program.

We are becoming increasingly aware of the limitations of "high tech" medicine in dealing with degenerative diseases, such as coronary heart disease, stroke, hypertension, diabetes, cancer and obesity. These killer diseases are *culturally conditioned* and *largely self-induced* by the way we live, particularly by the way we eat, drink, smoke and exercise. The scientific data is saying more clearly every day: "It is what we do, hour by hour, day by day, that largely determines the state of our health, whether we get sick, the disease we get, and perhaps even when we shall die."

The challenge of medicine today, as I see it, is to educate, motivate and inspire patients and public alike to replace their health-erosive lifestyle with a health-enhancing one.

Dr. Diehl, as a researcher, author, clinician and international lecturer, has done much in giving tens of thousands of people a clearer understanding of how they can contribute to their own health. He has provided them with the motivation to get started towards their recovery. As a gifted and dynamic communicator and scientist, he has given many the will and the skill to improve their lifestyle, so that they can stay younger longer and die younger *later* in life with genuine wellness and vitality. His goal is to help Americans die of a new cause of death: *of old age.*

It is my sincere hope that this book will extend his dedicated outreach. I know that many readers will reap great benefits as they follow these clinically proven and effective guidelines.

Charles Tam, M.D.
Director of Cardiology
St. Helena Hospital
Deer Park, CA 94576

To Your Health!

Here are the four fabulous diets—the "Monkey" diet, the "Baseball" diet, the "One-Hundred-Year-Old" diet, and the "Eat-Like-A-Horse" diet—you heard about on the television series "To Your Health," with Dr. Hans Diehl.

They aren't actual "diets," of course, but when you've tried almost every diet in the world and wound up irritable, disappointed, frustrated and fat, when you've eaten yourself sick, literally, and developed diabetes, high blood pressure, heart disease or one of the other all-American diet-related diseases—you don't need another "diet." You need a new dietary *lifestyle!*

All you have to do is combine a regular exercise program with a diet that is high in complex carbohydrates and fiber and low in fats, oils, cholesterol, sugar, and salt! That's it. That's all there is to it. But you could wind up in the doctor's office, or in the hospital, or worse if you don't follow the rules.

It's not a radical or new idea that your health, happiness, longevity and self-esteem, and your relationships with family, friends, and associates are all dependent on what and how you *eat*. The facts, studies, reports, and recommendations have been coming in for more than a decade. Then why haven't the government, the food industries, and the medical care system made a concerted effort to alert the public about our unhealthy eating habits? Are facts being kept from the public? Some people think so.

They say we're living longer these days, that advances in medical technology have increased our average life expectancy almost "30 years" since the turn of the century. *You'll see later that this figure is misleading.*[1] *But with the knowledge we have now, we could* and *should* live a healthy, happy 100 years!

To lead a long, strong and productive life, select food from the "four basic food groups," so they say. Not if you expect to live past middle age! The average American diet is killing us.

More than 4,000 times every day someone in the United States has a heart attack. A new diabetic is discovered every 50 seconds. And half the population over 40 years old has high blood pressure. Heart disease, cancer, high blood pressure, obesity, and diabetes are epidemic in America. It's a curious fact, however, that these chronic diseases are rarely found in 75 to 80 percent of the world's population!

Only Western industrialized societies like ours can afford diets that are rich in red meat, fish, poultry, eggs and processed food products loaded with sugar, oils, and salt. In America, 40 to 45 percent of the calories we eat come from fats, grease, and oil, with another 20 percent (38 teaspoons per day, per person) from sugar and related chemicals.

The consumption of fat, sugar and animal products has increased dramatically in this century. One hundred years ago Americans were far less dependent on animals to flesh out their diets. The meat they ate contained about one-half the amount of fat we enjoy today (and try to shed tomorrow). Fully 80 percent of the calories in a juicy sirloin steak are fat calories. In 1900 people got 70 percent of their protein from *plant* foods. Today we get 70 percent of our protein from *animal* products which are high in saturated fat and cholesterol.

A massive amount of research strongly suggests that our average American diet seriously undermines our health, limits our longevity and erodes our quality of life, especially in the last decades of life.[2] Despite the propaganda of powerful commercial food lobbies, Americans are becoming aware of the data and recalling the dictum they received from their grandmothers, "You are what you eat."

But it isn't easy to break old habits, to change your diet for life, even if it helps to break another bad habit we've acquired in this country—dying prematurely. The good news is that you don't have to give up good food OR good health. You can learn to enjoy more "foods as grown," simply prepared, without grease, sugar, and salt. Dig in, eat more potatoes, yams, squash, pasta, whole grain cereals, bread and brown rice—unrefined starchy foods that are low in calories and high in nutrients, along with plenty of fresh fruits and vegetables. Season your food with natural herbs and spices. Eating this way can help keep your wallet full, your silhouette slim, your arteries clean, and your mind and your body free from medications.

Our "To Your Health" TV series prompted thousands of requests, not for just another fad "diet of the month," but for some dietary guidelines that make sense for a plan to live well and die old with lots of good food and other good things in between. We share your concern and appreciate your requests. No matter what you call it, we dedicate the proven dietary plan that follows . . . To Your Health!

—LaVerne Tucker
President of The Quiet Hour, Inc.

---

[1] National Center for Health Statistics: *Vital Statistics of the U.S.,* Public Health Service. Hyattsville, MD. Sept. 26, 1985

[2] Hegsted DM (1977) Priorities in Nutrition in the U.S. *J Am Diet Assn* 71:9-12

1_____

What a Way to Go!

Candlelight, sparkling crystal, silver flanking china, a sommelier decanting wine from bottles draped in linen, fettucini in creamy cheese sauce, lime sorbet, marbled chateaubriand served with twice-fried potatoes and steamed broccoli drenched in hollandaise, white chocolate cheesecake with caramel sauce . . . brandy and cafe au lait!

It's our ideal, the "cuisine nonpareil," we aspire to even at the family dinner table. The image bespeaks affluence, the good life that American men and women have striven to build for themselves and their children for almost a century. Unfortunately this "good life" is not such a good life after all. If it were, then you might ask:

- Why do we spend more than one hundred million dollars annually for "magic pills" to help us lose weight, while the problem of obesity grows bigger every year?
- Why do half the people who die in the U. S. every year die prematurely of cardiovascular disease?
- Why is every third adult in this country attacked by heart disease, hypertension or stroke?

- Why are three out of four people killed by cardiovascular disease and cancer?

This isn't "nature's way." We haven't always died so massively of heart attacks, strokes, diabetes, and colon and breast cancer. Cardiovascular disease became rampant in America after World War I, when we began to afford diets rich in animal products and even more when the advertising and food industries found each other and persuaded us to eat a lot of unnatural, highly processed foods, crammed with calories and emptied of nutrition.[1]

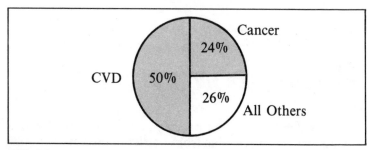

FIG. 1.1:
Causes of death in % of all deaths (US, 1985). 74% of deaths in the U.S. are caused by cardiovascular disease (CVC) and cancer.

It is a uniquely Western problem. People in China, Japan, and Southeast Asia seldom have many heart attacks. Most people in Africa and South and Central America have little fear of cancer or cardiovascular disease. Yet in North America, Australia, New Zealand, and affluent countries in Europe, heart disease and cancer are epidemic.

---

[1] Farquhar JW (1977) *The American Way of Life Need Not Be Hazardous to Your Health* New York W. N. Norton & Comp.

2

Promises, Profits & Prevarications

Despite magnificent medical centers, highly trained specialists and elaborate machinery, modern medicine is not very effective in dealing with these killer diseases.

For years we believed that with the right amount of money, research, manpower, and time, scientists could find a cure for everything. A futuristic Dr. McCoy would just press a metallic wand against our foreheads and off we'd fly into the universe cured of every earthly and alien disease in our body! It hasn't happened, and it probably won't. The main killers, cardiovascular disease and cancer, actually have mushroomed over the years. They're responsible for 74 percent of all deaths. (See Figure 2.1.) Our medical care system has become a salvage operation with doctors mostly treating the victims. What is needed, we are learning, is a lifestyle approach that can largely *prevent* these diseases and, in many cases, *reverse* their effects.

Coronary bypass surgery, for instance, is not proving to be the hoped-for answer for victims of heart attacks. Last year nearly 250,000 bypasses were performed in the hope that the surgery would prolong life by preventing recurrent heart attacks. But for most people, taking a vein from the

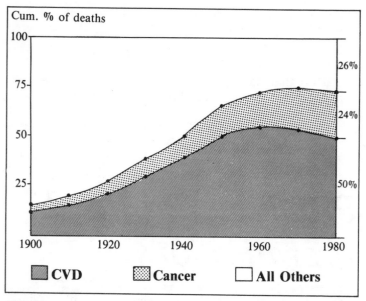

FIG. 2.1:
Mortality Trends for CVD and Cancer (US, 1900-1985)
Cardiovascular disease (CVD) and cancer (as a percentage of all causes of death) have increased over the years. While CVD at the turn of the century accounted for 10-15%, it now accounts for every second death. Similar increases are shown for cancer, which is continuing to rise despite heroic after-the-fact medical interventions.

leg and using it to bypass a blocked or damaged artery in the heart doesn't solve the problem. Veins are anatomically weaker than arteries and can suffer the same effects of cardiovascular disease when they are used to replace arteries. In fact, 15 to 30 percent of the grafted veins close within twelve months of surgery. At about $50,000 per operation, bypass surgery does improve the quality of life for some people, but not always. If a victim's grafts close or a second heart attack strikes, another bypass may be performed; but surgery is often only a stay of execution unless substantial changes in lifestyle, especially in the area of diet, are implemented to keep the implanted veins open and healthy.

As a society we have developed an almost blind faith in

medical technology and drug therapy, strengthened by too many TV episodes like those of Drs. Kildare and Ben Casey! We've devised two basic problem-solving techniques—surgery and medications. Let's look at medication.

More than half of cardiovascular patients wind up taking prescription drugs that don't cure—they just alleviate symptoms.

Diuretic drugs (water pills), commonly prescribed for high blood pressure, actually *contribute* to heart disease by elevating cholesterol levels, and they *contribute* to diabetes by increasing blood sugar levels. Norman Kaplan, M.D., a recognized authority on the treatment of hypertension, warned in *Hospital Tribune,* May 16, 1985, "No single hypertensive agent has more adverse effects than diuretics. The benefits do not outweigh the risks, especially in older patients." Yet last year nearly four hundred million dollars worth of the most commonly prescribed diuretic drug, *Dyazide,* was sold in the U.S. (See Chapter 7).

Several prescription drugs used to lower cholesterol have proved to be more dangerous than therapeutic. As a result of the six-year Coronary Drug Project conducted by the National Institutes of Health and published in 1975, two of the then commonly prescribed drugs were abruptly taken off the market when the study showed that more people died in the group taking the drugs than in the group taking "sugar pills"—placebos![3]

A six-year investigation of the cholesterol lowering drug *Atromid-S* showed no decrease in coronary deaths. In fact, there was an increase in mortality among patients taking *Atromid-S* because of resulting diseases of the liver, gall bladder, and intestines. The drug had serious pathological and, occasionally, lethal side effects. But in 1985 more than a million *Atromid-S* prescriptions were written—despite this warning from the National Institutes of Health in 1978: "The use of these cholesterol lowering drugs should be deferred until distinct benefits are demonstrated and significant toxicity can be excluded."[4]

Drugs are no help at all in preventing or reversing coronary artery disease. They may relieve some of the

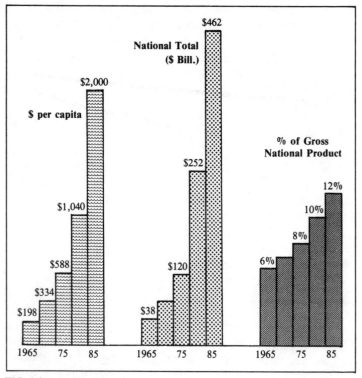

FIG. 2.2:
Medical Expenditures over the past 20 years have skyrocketed: our annual national bill is now exceeding $500 billion, which amounts to $2,000 for every man, woman and child, and the percentage of our earnings paid for medical care has gone from 6% to 12%.

symptoms, they may make the electrocardiogram look better, but the disease keeps progressing and killing 750,000 Americans every year!

It's an expensive way to go. In 1965 we spent thirty-eight billion dollars for medical care: 5.9 percent of all our earnings went to pay medical bills. This year the bill will be closer to five hundred billion, or 12 percent of our total earnings. It averages out to $2,000 per person every year for medical care, and these increases are being reflected in our skyrocketing health insurance premiums. (See Figure 2.2)

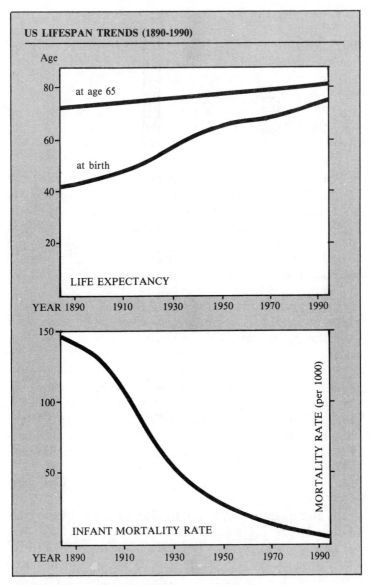

FIG. 2.3: U.S. LIFESPAN TRENDS
Life expectancy at birth is increasing. However, during the past 100 years the life expectancy for 65 year-olds has increased only marginally.

The construction of a new hospital costs $300,000 per bed! Sixty percent of the cost goes for medical equipment that becomes obsolete in less than a decade. Medical care is the second biggest business in the country—second only to— are you ready for this—the food industry!

All this money, energy, research and equipment has yielded precious little in the way of better health. And spending twice as much will not add significantly to our life span if it is directed mainly to symptomatic and salvage operations.

For years we have cherished the belief that we are the world's healthiest society. Our life expectancy statistics prove it, don't they? Not really. We know that a baby born in 1987 has a life expectancy 27 years greater than that of a baby born at the turn of the century. But the statistics are based on dramatically reduced mortality rates of newborns and children. Improvements in public health and sanitation, rather than heroic advances in medical science, deserve most of the credit for this. Sadly, a sixty-five-year-old American today has about the same number of years to look forward to as his counterpart did eighty-seven years ago (See Fig. 2.3).[5]

In today's world our health is not determined by the doctor's intellect or training or the size of the hospital, but by our individual lifestyles, our physiological inheritance, and our physical environment. Good health is largely the result of what we are willing to do for ourselves and by how we choose to live, especially in the matter of eating, drinking, smoking, and exercise.

Bibliography—Chapter 2

[1] Rahimtoola SH (1982) Coronary Bypass Surgery for Chronic Angina—1981. *Circulation* 65:225-241

[2] Coronary Artery Surgery Study. (1983) A randomized trial of coronary artery bypass surgery. *Circulation* 68:939-960

[3] Coronary Drug Project Research Group (1975) Clofibrate and niacin in coronary heart disease. *JAMA* 231:360-381

[4] Rifkind BM and RI Levy (1978) Testing the Lipid hypothesis. *Arch Surg* 113:80-83

[5] National Center for Health Statistics: *Vital Statistics of the U.S.* Public Health Service. Hyattsville, MD. Sept. 26, 1985

Atherosclerosis: The Silent Killer

In kindergarten we learn that pain is a warning that something is wrong in our body, and we grow up heeding these warnings. Unfortunately, the first sign that something is wrong with our arteries is often *sudden death*. The trouble usually begins in childhood, and it usually develops slowly over the years, sometimes taking fifty years to make itself known, sometimes less!

The trouble is **atherosclerosis,** hardening of the arteries, the underlying cause of most cardiovascular disease.

You were born with clean, flexible arteries, and they should stay that way until you die of that rare disease called Old Age. However, the arteries in most Americans are clogging up with cholesterol, fats, and calcium—a concoction that hardens in time and finally chokes arteries completely. Deprived of oxygenated blood, the heart has an attack, the brain has a stroke, and the victim has a bypass, or physical therapy, or . . .! All too often, there is no warning!

This shortage of oxygen (hypoxia) due to atherosclerosis is the cause of various hypoxic diseases affecting the circulatory system in different critical areas:

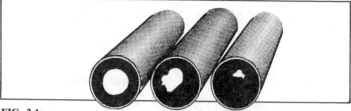

FIG. 3.1:
Atherosclerosis, once thought to be a degenerative disorder, is a progressive narrowing of the arteries throughout the body, which is fed by rich diets, high in cholesterol and fats and aggravated by smoking and high blood pressure. Cholesterol, fats and other materials accumulate in the arterial wall forming plaques, which in due time can disrupt and interrupt vital blood flow.

Angina Pectoris: The flow of oxygenated blood to the heart muscle itself is impeded or temporarily blocked, causing pain in the chest, in the left arm, or between the shoulder blades.

Myocardial Infarction (Heart Attack): A part of the heart muscle becomes starved for oxygen and dies.

Intermittent Claudication: Restricted flow of oxygenated blood to the leg muscles causes acute pain and cramps, until the person stops his activity and the blood begins to flow again through the narrowed femoral arteries.

Gangrene: Body tissue, usually in the toes and feet, decays and dies due to lack of blood, usually necessitating amputation.

Impotence: The inability to deliver adequate blood to the organ on demand and on a sustained basis. In 50 to 60 percent of the cases, atherosclerosis is the underlying cause.

Hypertension: Greater force is necessary to push blood through narrowed vessels to supply body oxygen needs, hence high blood pressure.

Cerebral Infarction (Stroke): Brittle, narrowed arteries in or leading to the brain rupture or plug up, causing paralysis or sudden death.

Senility: An inadequate supply of oxygen to vital brain tissue is believed to cause this debilitating disorder in 40 to 50 percent of the cases.

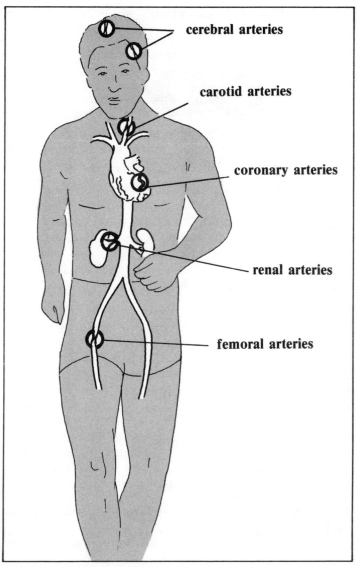

FIG. 3.2: Atherosclerotic Sites
Atherosclerotic plaques most commonly involve the coronary, carotid and cerebral arteries affecting bloodflow and oxygen delivery to the heart muscle and to brain structures. Plaques can also interfere with proper bloodflow to the kidneys and the legs by affecting the renal and femoral arteries.

Hearing Loss: Loss of hearing, especially in the high frequency range, may be caused by atherosclerosis.

Visual Loss: Tunnel vision and retinal detachment are processes associated with inadequate blood flow.

Cancer: Some of the common cancers may be related to inadequate oxygenation of vital tissues due to atherosclerosis. It is intriguing that cancers of the breast, prostate, and colon are mainly found in societies afflicted with cardiovascular disease.[1]

It may come as a surprise, but there simply aren't any symptoms or signs of trouble until a person's arteries are about 80 percent closed. Dr. Kuller, who conducted the Sudden Death Study in Baltimore, found that 24 percent of the heart attack victims in the study had seen their physician in the week preceding the attack, and most had received a clean bill of health.[2]

The disease usually begins to develop in the pre-teen years in our society, and most attacks occur before the age of sixty-five. Autopsies revealed that three-quarters of the American soldiers who died in the Korean conflict had already significantly narrowed coronary arteries. Their average age was twenty-two.[3, 4]

Every year hundreds of thousands of people die of heart attacks and other hypoxic diseases without a murmur of protest from the public, the press, or government agencies. Such a rash of killings by any other means would mobilize the country! Atherosclerosis is not a "natural" way to go; it's not the inevitable result of the aging process. Large populations in the world are unaffected by it. It's those of us who consume large amounts of cholesterol and excessive fats, especially animal fats, that are targets for the "silent killer."

Ultimate solutions will not be found in the present medical care system or in the ministrations of doctors during and after an attack. Only *you* can slow down the atherosclerosis process, stop it, and reverse its effects!

What Causes Atherosclerosis?

The mystery of atherosclerosis began to unravel when Russian researchers around the turn of the century found that rabbits fed a diet of meat and eggs developed high levels of cholesterol and severely clogged arteries.[5]

Then in 1916 a Dutch researcher in Indonesia reported that Javanese people had very low cholesterol levels and were virtually free of atherosclerosis in contrast to people living in Holland. When he noticed that Javanese stewards working—and eating—on Dutch steamships developed the same high cholesterol levels as did the Hollanders, he suggested that atherosclerosis might not be related to race but to diet.[6]

Additional support for the "diet" theory was found during World War II when most Europeans were forced to change their eating habits from their customary diet of meat, eggs, and dairy products to a more austere diet of potatoes, grains, beans, roots, and vegetables. For nearly a decade a substantial decrease in atherosclerosis was documented in various European populations.[7] Finland, deprived of meat and butterfat as a result of the Russian invasion, experienced a sharp drop in atherosclerosis.[8] Norway and Sweden "suffered" a similar fate dut to Nazi occupation. In Belgium Dr. William Castelli and other pathologists had a difficult time finding atherosclerosed arteries to show medical students.

"There was an incredibly severe decline in coronary heart disease," Dr. Castelli recalls, "because the Nazis had taken away the livestock, and most of the people were living on potatoes and bread." [9]

The most unusual evidence came from Nazi concentration camps. Despite subhuman diets and torture, survivors of the Holocaust were surprisingly free of atherosclerosis. It was the first indication—later confirmed by angiographic examinations of American POW's in Vietnam—that the process of atherosclerosis is reversible. Those who were held the longest in captivity had the cleanest arteries.

Bibliography—Chapter 3

[1] Marvick C. (1986) A Nation of Jack Sprats? Cholesterol Program to Stress Dietary Changes. *JAMA* 256:2775-2779

[2] Kuller Lewis et al (1966) Epidemiological Study of Sudden Deaths Due to Atherosclerotic Heart Disease. *Circulation* 34:1056-1068

[3] Enos WF et al (1953) Coronary Disease Among U.S. Soldiers Killed in Action in Korea. *JAMA* 152:1090-1093

[4] Strong JP (1986) Coronary Atherosclerosis in Soldiers. *JAMA* 256:2863-2866

[5] Anitschkow N (1913) Ueber Experimentelle Cholesterin Steatose und ihre Bedeutung for die Entstehung einiger pathologischer Prozesse. *Zbl Path* 26:1-8

[6] DeLanger CD (1916) Cholesterol Metabolism in Racial Pathology. *Geneesk Tydschr Nederl Indie* 56:1-34

[7] Malmros H (1950) The relation of nutrition to health. *Acta Med Scand* Suppl. 246:128-139

[8] Vartiainen I and K Kanerva (1947) Arteriosclerosis in Wartime. *Ann Intern Med* (Finland) 536:748-758

[9] Castelli W (1986) personal communication

4

The Risk Factor Concept

In 1947 Dr. Ancel Keys began a study at the University of Minnesota in which 281 businessmen in their forties and fifties were selected for a fifteen-year study of heart disease. When the medical records of the men who suffered coronary events during the study period were compared with those of men who did not, Dr. Keys found three big differences: the heart attack victims had higher blood cholesterols, higher blood pressures, and more of them smoked, putting them, Dr. Keys surmised, at greater risk for heart disease.

About that time (1949), the famous Framingham Study[2] (which is still in progress) was initiated, in which 5,209 men and women between the ages of thirty and sixty were enlisted in a "life and death" study of cardiovascular disease. The participants have lived in a scientific "fish bowl"—their habits, physical characteristics, histories (medical and otherwise) and laboratory tests are carefully assessed to see if they relate to the development of various circulatory diseases. The researchers in this monumental study, under the present leadership of Dr. William Castelli, have found the following:

1. Fifty-year-old men with blood cholesterols over 295 mg% are 9 times more likely to develop

atherosclerosis than men the same age with cholesterols under 200.

2. Smokers are 10 times more likely to die by age 60 than non-smokers.

3. Men 20 percent overweight are 5 times more likely to die of cardiovascular disease by age 60 than are men of normal weight.

4. Every second death is due to heart disease or stroke.

5. By age 60, one out of every five men has had a heart attack.

6. By age 50, every third person has high blood pressure and is 3 times more likely to die of cardiovascular disease than is a person with normal blood pressure.

The Framingham Study confirmed Dr. Keys' "Risk Factor" concept in determining the likelihood of cardiovascular disease and made it as important as the germ theory is to the infectious diseases. What are *your* chances of having a heart attack? Look at the risks you're taking.

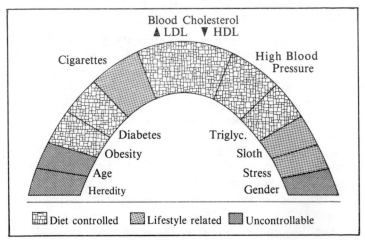

FIG. 4.1: Risk Factors in Heart Disease
Note: (1) The higher on the arch, the higher the contribution of the risk factor to CVD. (2) Five of the eight controllable risk factors are mostly under the control of diet.

The higher on the arch, the more important and consequential the risk. Therefore, high cholesterol (especially LDL cholesterol), high blood pressure and smoking are major risk factors. Any combination of risks only magnifies the problem. And the longer you wait to change your lifestyle, the more likely you are to develop heart disease (or one of the other hypoxic diseases). *Atherosclerosis is a loaded gun, and time pulls the trigger!*

Some low risk factors, such as age, gender, and heredity, are beyond our control. Women are somewhat protected against heart disease until menopause, compared with men the same age. And only one person in 500 is really "programmed" genetically for heart disease.

Fortunately, the majority of risk factors in heart disease are controllable. You can modify your cholesterol, blood pressure, triglycerides, obesity, and diabetes simply by changing your diet. You can control or learn to cope with stress, give up smoking, and start a rational program of daily physical activity. Well, some cynics may ask, "What kind of life is that?" These measures can dramatically improve your chances of avoiding atherosclerosis related diseases. The fact is you can clean out your arteries, stop dying of atherosclerosis, and extend your active, productive years. You can change your risk factors, no matter how old you are, often in just a few weeks. People who are doing this are happy and feeling good, and are leading busy and fulfilling lives.

Personal Health Improvement

By examining the risk factors you can estimate your chances of developing heart disease. And by modifying the risk factors, you can improve your chances of avoiding a heart attack. Notice the contrast in Table 4.1.

As you can see, our man "A" is 140 times more likely to develop heart disease than his healthy contemporary is. If "A" were 45 years old, he would have a 32 percent chance of developing heart disease within six years. If he were 55, his chances would be almost 50-50. In other words, as we

Risk Factor	Male "A"	Male "B"
Cholesterol (mg%)	310	150
Blood Pressure	160/90	110/75
Smoking	yes	no
EKG	positive	negative
Diabetes	yes	no
Risk of Developing Heart Disease within 6 years	**14%**	**0.1%**

TABLE 4.1:
Risk of Developing Heart Disease within six years according to Presence of Risk Factors (man, age 35 years)
Because of the difference in the presence of risk factors, subject "A" has a 14% chance of developing heart disease, subject "B" only .1%.

get older, our chances of escaping heart disease get slimmer.

Multimillion dollar studies funded by the National Institutes of Health have shown that 63 to 80 percent of all major coronary events before age 65 could be prevented if Americans would lower their cholesterol (under 180), lower their blood pressure (under 125), and quit smoking.[3,4] These simple changes in lifestyle would do more to improve the health of our nation than would all the hospitals, surgeries, and drugs combined.

The Heart Screen Test

The Risk Factor concept is an important tool in helping you determine if, why, and when you might have a heart attack.[5,6] And the presence of multiple risk factors is also the major determinant of graft closure after bypass surgery.[7] It's worth taking the Heart Screen test!

The Risk Factor concept is an important tool is helping your determine if, why, and when you might have a heart attack. And the presence of multiple risk factors is also the major determinant of graft closure after bypass surgery. It's worth taking the Heart Screen test!

The Heart Screen test will approximate your relative risk and will help you to identify areas that you may want to work on and to set goals. In this self-scoring test (adapted from several large studies), eight risk factors are listed and scores of zero to eight are assigned to each factor.

You may want to skip to pages 32-34 at the end of this chapter to take the test before you read on.

If you've taken the Heart Screen Test and scored somewhat higher than ideal, here's a word of encouragement: **Eat!** Matter of fact, eat your way to a lower score, **eat your way back to health.** Eat more—and lose weight! If you think we've gone a little too far this time and that it's impossible to eat more than you ever have before and still lose weight, remember the "Eat Like a Horse Diet" we recommended on TV. We weren't kidding—well, maybe a little.

Bibliography—Chapter 4

[1] Keys A et al (1963) Coronary Heart Disease Among Minnesota Business and Professional Men Followed 15 Years. *Circulation* 28:381-395

[2] The Framingham Study (1973) (Eds) Kannel WB and T. Gordon DHEW Public. # (NIH) 74-618

[3] Byington R et al (1979) Recent Trends of Major Coronary Risk Factors and CHD Mortality in the US. *in* Proceedings of the Conference on the Decline in CHD Mortality. (Eds) Havlik RJ and M. Feinlieb. US Dept. HELJ, PHS # (NIH) 79-1610

[4] Stamler J et al (1986) Is Relationship Between Serum Cholesterol and Risk of Premature Death From Coronary Heart Disease Continuous and Graded? *JAMA* 256:2823-2828

[5] Cooper T (1981) The Scientific Foundation for the Prevention of Coronary Heart Disease (Keynote address) *Am J Card* 47:720-724

[6] Gohlke H et al (1980) Myocardial Infarction at Young Age—Correlation of Angiographic Findings with Risk Factors and History in 619 Patients. *Circulation II* 62:4

[7] Barndt R et al (1981) Serial Angiographic Correlations of Progression and Regression of Atherosclerosis with Risk Factor Levels. *Arteriosclerosis* 1:1-8

TABLE 4.1: Heart Screen
Self Scoring Test of Heart Attack and Stroke Risk

	Risk Level and Score		
Risk Factor	**0**	**1**	**2**
1. Cholesterol* (mg %)	under 160	160-179	180-199
2. Blood Pressure* (mmHg)	under 110	110-119	120-129
3. Smoking (cig./day)	none	up to 5	5-9
4. Overweight** (in %)	0-4%	5-9%	10-14%
5. Trigylcerides* (mg %)	under 100	100-149	150-249
6. Diabetes (duration)	None	under 5 years	5-10 years
7. Resting Pulse beats/min.	under 56	56-62	63-69
8. Stress	Rarely tense	Tense 3x/wk	Tense 2-3x/day

* To determine your cholesterol, triglycerides and blood pressure, just see your physician. The blood test is very simple, inexpensive, takes about five minutes, and it will tell you a lot!

TABLE 4.1: Heart Screen (continued)
Self Scoring Test of Heart Attack and Stroke Risk

Risk Level and Score					
3	**4**	**5**	**6**	**7**	**8**
200-219	220-239	240-259	260-279	280-299	300 plus
130-139	140-159	160 plus			
10-19	20-29	30 +			
15-19%	20-29%	30% +			
250-349	350 +				
10 + years					
70-80	80 +				
Tense & rushed	on tranquilizers				

Risk Factor	Score
Cholesterol	
Blood Pressure	
Smoking	
Overweight	
Triglycerides	
Diabetes	
Pulse	
Stress	
Total Score:	

** To determine your percentage of overweight, look up your ideal weight on page 39 (Stanford formula) and subtract it from your actual weight. Divide the difference in pounds by your ideal weight and multiply by 100.

How to interpret your Heart Screen Score

(Total Score)

0-6 Ideal: Development of heart disease or stroke is extremely unlikely, especially if cholesterol level is below 180. People in this category make good role models and teachers for those who are striving towards this very risk zone.

7-14 Elevated Risk: The development of heart disease or stroke is about one-third of the U.S. average.

15-22 High Risk: This is the American average. You *cannot* afford to be average!

23-30 Very High Risk: The development of heart disease and stroke is about three times the U.S. average. Action is imperative! You may be able to drop 4 to 6 points within 4 to 8 weeks by lowering cholesterol and blood pressure through dietary change.

31-38 Dangerous!!!!!: The likelihood of having a heart attack or stroke is about 4 to 6 times the U.S. average! Or about 50 times higher than the Ideal group. Set goals and go into action without delay. Drop 4 to 6 points within 4 to 6 weeks by making some lifestyle changes!

5

Obesity: A Slim View of a Broad Subject

After twenty years of dieting, says a national survey, the average American is now five pounds **heavier.** Some diet! One out of every two adults in the U.S. is overweight. The American Seating Company, one of the world's leading chair manufacturers, claims their standard seats had to be widened two inches to accommodate the ever expanding American derrière—no joke!

Obesity (by definition, you're **obese** if you're at least twenty percent overweight) is one of the leading public health problems in America. So severe is this disease that 34 million Americans are at serious medical risk. Their chances of

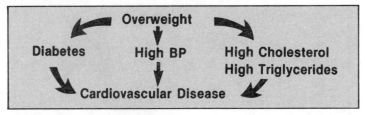

FIG. 5.1:
Relationship of Obesity to CVD
Obesity contributes directly to development of CVD, and by influencing CVD-risk factors.

having heart disease is three times greater than those of people of normal weight. They are five times more likely to develop diabetes, five times more likely to have higher than average cholesterol, six times more likely (especially women) to develop gall bladder disease. And they are more likely to develop cancer of the colon, rectum, prostate, breast, cervix, uterus and ovaries and to develop osteoarthritis and low-back pain. To put it mildly, being twenty percent or more overweight is not healthy.

According to recent reports from the Framingham Study, even 5 to 10 pounds of extra weight is associated with higher mortality rates; i.e. almost any degree of overweight has an adverse effect on health and longevity. Every extra pound shaves about one month from your lifespan; 60 pounds overweight, for instance, will cost you 5 years!

Our self image also suffers. Obesity is a great psychological burden, especially in our slim-oriented society.

Feeding the Life

It isn't true that you will just naturally gain weight as you get older (most people gain about one pound per year after

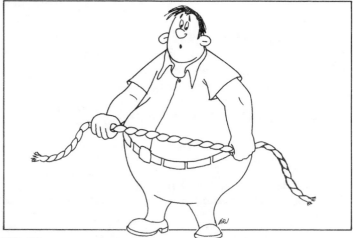

FIG. 5.2:
The longer the WAISTLINE, **the shorter** the LIFELINE.

age twenty). And it isn't your fault if you're overweight.

Our culture is the culprit! Our magazines are filled with beautiful, slender people—and recipes for fattening foods. The food we eat at home and the foods offered at dinner parties, in restaurants, and even in hospitals, contribute to our obesity. Our idea of elegant dining is conducive to romance—and coronary infarction.

Our knee-jerk reaction to overweight is to go on a diet. Too many people fall prey to the "merchants of misery" who offer quick fixes through quack remedies and semi-starvation plans. A recent survey commissioned by the Calorie Control Council found that 40 to 50 percent of Americans between 35 and 59 years old were dieting.

In addition to being unappetizing and monotonous, "grapefruit" diets, "prune juice" diets, "high protein" diets and the like can be harmful to your health, your wealth, and your self respect. Stay away from them. Let **diets** die. Instead, adopt a sound, rational dietary plan for **better health.**

If you don't modify your lifestyle and choose the right food on a regular basis, the weight you lose on any diet will come right back. Almost 95 percent of all dieters regain their

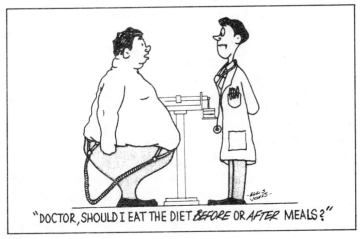

"DOCTOR, SHOULD I EAT THE DIET *BEFORE* OR *AFTER* MEALS?"

FIG. 5.3:
Let Diets Die!

lost weight within a year and have to diet all over again. Constantly losing and gaining weight is frustrating and demoralizing. It often leaves serious psychological scars. The *rhythm method of girth control* just doesn't work.

Some dieters even flirt with death. The "Last Chance Diet," a liquid protein concoction designed to lose weight fast, was the last diet 58 people ever tried—they died. The "Cambridge Diet" was implicated in several deaths and had to be revamped. For good reasons most diet plans warn against staying too long on a diet and suggest "doctor's supervision."

Over the years the medical establishment has tried many drugs, among them appetite suppressants, amphetamines, diuretics, hormones, and Vitamin B12 injections. Over one hundred million dollars worth were sold last year. But diet drugs have not only proved worthless, they're often downright dangerous. Many have serious side effects, some are addictive, and perhaps most important, they all delay and discourage the adoption of healthy and effective dietary lifestyles.

Inevitably surgical procedures have been tried, such as intestinal bypass, stomach stapling, jaw-wiring, and lipectomy (suctioning fat from under the skin with a vacuum device). At $15,000 each, the *intestinal* bypass seemed marvelously successful at first until people began to develop kidney stones, bone disease, incapacitating diarrhea, anemia, and liver disease, and many died. The operation was soon outlawed. The latest wrinkle is "balloon implantation," in which a balloon is inserted in the stomach and then inflated. The patient feels full, eats less, loses weight—and gains it back once more when the balloon is removed, thus bursting another bubble of technological wizardry.

The secret of success is to adopt a *dietary lifestyle* that will keep you healthy, give you more energy, lower your risk of heart disease, stroke, and cancer, reduce your food bill, allow you to eat as much as you want, and still lose one or two pounds a week without ever being hungry. Impossible? Read on.

Who's Fat Anyway?

The Stanford Heart Disease Prevention Program uses this simple formula to determine your "ideal" weight:

> Women: Height in inches x 3.5 pounds minus 108
> Men: Height in inches x 4.0 pounds minus 128
> (Large-boned adults add 8 percent; small-boned adults subtract 4 percent)

Metropolitan Life Insurance Company tables (see next page) are based on the results of a study by the Society of Actuaries, pooling the experience of twenty-six U.S. and Canadian life insurance companies over a period of twenty years.

Since obesity has been defined as "a pathological condition characterized by an accumulation of fat in excess of that necessary for optimum function," a more accurate measurement can be determined by hydrostatic weighing—or by the simple "pinch-an-inch" test. (If you can pinch an inch of fat at your lower rib, you're overweight.)

Did you hear the one about the woman who was so fat she had to let out her mirrors . . .?! A full-length mirror can tell you if you're fat. But not why. Why are Americans, on the average, heavier than the citizens of any other major nation?

One study of obesity shows a genetic link, while another indicates a strong environmental influence, noting that fat people usually have fat spouses, fat children and even fat pets! Twenty years ago, Dr. Jules Hirsch from Rockefeller University, suggested that obesity could be related to being overfed during the first two years of life, thus creating billions of extra fat cells that in adulthood are resistant to weight loss. Others say personality factors are the cause of the problem. And two percent of the obese population can blame an underfunctioning thyroid gland.

The various theories are fascinating to academicians and researchers who make a living studying them. However, for most of us the basic cause of excess weight is this: we eat more calories than we burn up!

Overweight occurs when food calories exceed the energy

HEIGHT (Without Shoes)	WEIGHT IN LBS.*		
	Small Frame	Medium Frame	Large Frame
MEN+			
5'2"	115-123	121-133	129-144
4"	121-129	127-139	135-152
6"	128-137	134-147	142-161
8"	136-145	142-156	151-170
10"	144-154	150-165	159-179
6'0"	152-162	158-175	168-189
2"	160-171	167-185	178-199
4"	168-179	177-195	187-209
WOMEN+			
4'10"	96-104	101-113	109-125
5'0"	102-110	107-119	115-131
2"	108-116	113-126	121-138
4"	114-123	120-135	129-146
6"	122-131	128-143	137-154
8"	130-140	136-151	145-163
10"	138-148	144-159	153-173

Ideal Weights according to Frame

[1] Adapted from Metropolitan Life Insurance Corporation Tables, 1959.[2]

[2] The 1959 table has been recognized by many prominent researchers, including Dr. Castelli from the Framingham Study, as being more representative of ideal weights than the revised 1983 chart.

* Includes one lb. for ordinary indoor clothing.

+ Age 25 years and older.

requirement of the body for physical activity and metabolism. We "burn up" food to produce heat and perform muscular activities. Weight stays the same if we completely utilize all our food for fuel and maintenance.

But excess calories are stored as fat (triglycerides). It makes no difference whether they come from sugar, protein, starch, or fat. If the calories are not used, they will be deposited in our "fat bank," and this bank tends to set up branch offices, embarrassingly, in and around our midsection. *For each deposit of 3,500 calories, we earn one pound of fat.* Just an extra 100 calories a day can mean 10 pounds in a year. Not a bad investment—for a whale.

For the rest of us, if you cut your food intake by only 500 calories a day for seven days, at the end of the week you'll have lost one pound of fat!

To effect such a negative energy balance, where you burn more calories than you take in, you have three options:

Option #1: Decrease food calories; maintain activity level.

Option #2: Maintain food calories; increase activity level.

Option #3: Decrease food calories; increase activity level.

The most effective option is #3, which gives you a win-win situation: you take in fewer calories and burn more through exercise.

But we're suggesting a way to **in**crease the amount of food you eat while **de**creasing calories! *You can eat all you like* of the right kind of nutritious foods (you'll soon like them all), and still lose 1-2 pounds a week especially if you put your best food forward and walk at least 30 minutes every day.

Grandma Was Right!

Food just isn't the same as it was eighty-five or a hundred years ago—for many reasons. Before the turn of the century, the American diet consisted mostly of foods "as grown," mostly in local gardens and nearby farms. It was supplemented with a few staples from the General Store and some meat from range-fed cattle. Our great-grandparents didn't have 15,000 slickly packaged, cleverly promoted products waiting at the local supermarket, or 60,000 fast food restaurants spending more than one billion dollars advertising "take-out" service (nutrition is what they "take out"). Families ate their freshly cooked food and home-baked bread around their own tables.

But times and tastes have changed. We spend 40 percent of our food dollars "eating out." Our livestock are fattened in feedlots where lack of exercise, antibiotics, and "growth enhancers" produce bigger cattle faster and juicier meat with about twice the fat as range-fed cattle. Farm   produce is processed, refined, concentrated, sugared, salted, and chemically engineered to produce taste sensations which are rich in calories but poverty stricken in nutritional value. Advertising and mass marketing have created a demand that produces big profit margins and fat bodies.

Food-as-grown is nutritionally balanced. However, refinement strips food of most of its fiber and nutrients. Processing adds calories, subtracts nutrition, and contributes myriads of chemical additives. Strip seven pounds of sugar beets of their bulk, fiber, and nutrients for instance, and you get one pound of "pure" sugar!

The modern shift away from complex carbohydrates (whole plant foods, rich in fiber) to more animal products and processed foods has adversely affected the health and nutrition of the American people.

In 1860 nutritionally rich complex carbohydrates (whole grain bread and cereal, potatoes, beans, and vegetables) accounted for 53 percent of people's caloric intake. Today these starchy foods represent only 22 percent of our daily

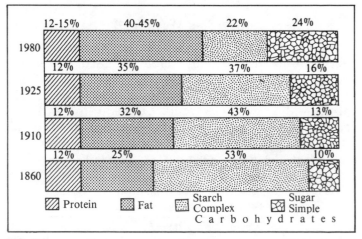

FIG. 5.4:
Dietary Trends (in % of total calories) US 1860-1980
The American diet has been shifting, resulting in a dramatic change in diet composition, where now more calories come from sugar (simple carbohydrates) than from starch (complex carbohydrates) and almost half the calories come from fat.

calories, whereas fat consumption since the turn of the century has almost doubled and sugar intake has increased by 240 percent!

Our diet has changed dramatically. Hot, whole grain cereals like oatmeal have been replaced at the breakfast table by cold, pre-sweetened flakes. Lunch typically consists of French fries slathered with ketchup, a hamburger, and soda. Supper, likely as not, comes frozen in a cardboard box. Between meals there are Zingers, Ding-Dongs, chips, and donuts.

Things were different in the old days. Grandma knew that food, not clothes, makes the man (or woman). Naked, empty calories, stripped of their fiber and nutrients, can't build healthy children and energetic adults, but they can put bulges on bodies that no seamstress can hide. "You are what you eat," she warned us solemnly.

Running on Empty Calories

Fifty percent of the American diet is made up of processed, concentrated calories, devoid of vital nutrients and valuable fiber, that get you nowhere but overweight.

SUGAR and other refined sweeteners account for 21 percent of our daily calories. That amounts to 142 pounds of sugar a year, ¾ cup, or 38 teaspoons a day for every man, woman and child.

Many of us aren't aware of the amount of sugar we eat

Empty Calories	As % of total cal.
Sugar	21%
Visible fats and oils	20%
Alcohol	9%
Total Empty Calories	50%

TABLE 5.1:
U.S. Diet—Empty Calories as % of total calories eaten
Half of the calories eaten by Americans are virtually devoid of vitamins, minerals, fiber, but loaded with calories. No wonder that many are OVERFED and UNDERNOURISHED.

Sugar Content in Selected Drinks	
Brand (12 oz.)	**Teaspoons of sugar**
Tang	12
Coke	11
Mountain Dew	11
Pepsi	10
Kool-Aid	9
Sprite	9

TABLE 5.2

because much of it is hidden. (See Appendix, page 197)

1. Soft drinks and fruit-flavored drinks hide the most. Americans now drink more soda than water, about 50 gallons per person per year.

2. Bakery goods and milk products hide their share of sugar. One piece of chocolate cake contains 15 teaspoonsfull; one cup of frozen yogurt has 12 teaspoons; one cup of chocolate pudding or ice cream has 6 to 8 teaspoons.

3. Sweets, such as candies, syrups, jellies, jams, and gelatin represent the largest source of sugar consumed by people over 35 years old. *Jello,* for instance, is 83 percent sugar.

4. Ready-to-eat cereals are often loaded with sugar. Hidden inside the average box of pre-sweetened cereal, cleverly disguised with cartoons and special offers, is up to ½ pound of sugar. A two-ounce serving of Kellogg's *Honey Smacks* hides 8 teaspoons of sugar; *Apple Jacks, Froot Loops, Super Golden Crisp* and *Boo Berry* are more than 50 percent sugar!

Cooked, whole grain cereals, rich in fiber expand in your stomach giving a sensation of fullness, and they save you money (how sweet that is). On the other hand, sugary cereals crumble and shrink almost to nothing, and they're expensive. (See Table 5.3)

The least nutritious foods with the most sugar are the most widely advertised. At a Senate sub-committee meeting, the president of Tufts University, Dr. Jean Mayer, stated: "The enormous resources of advertising go far toward the destruction of our more sensible (eating) habits."

Effect of Food Processing on Price.

Natural Cereal	Cost
½ lb. rolled oats	$0.30
½ lb. seven-grain cereal	$0.42

Processed Cereal	Cost
½ lb. refined wheat (in 18 oz. of *Honey Smacks*)	$2.80

TABLE 5.3

Sugar is found nearly everywhere: in canned soups, pot pies, TV dinners, even in bouillon. Consumer Union found *Hot Cocoa Mix* to be 82 percent sugar; *Coffeemate,* 65 percent; *Shake 'N Bake Barbeque Style,* 51 percent; *Heinz Ketchup,* 30 percent; *Hamburger Helper,* 23 percent; *Cool Whip,* 21 percent; etc., etc., etc. And sugar by any other name—sucrose, dextrose, glucose, lactose, maltose, fructose, honey, corn syrup, and molasses—is still sugar, calorie rich, nutrition poor, and fattening.

VISIBLE FATS AND OILS make up another 20 percent of our daily calories. Cooking and salad oils, shortening, mayonnaise, butter, and margarine, for instance, are all very low in nutritional value and very high in calories. In fact,

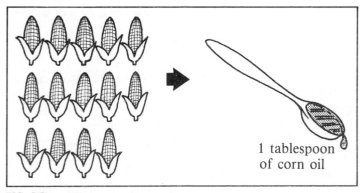

1 tablespoon of corn oil

FIG. 5.5:
Food Refinement leads to Calorie Concentration

ounce for ounce, fats are twice as fattening as sugar! There are nine calories in one gram of fat. There are only four calories in a gram of carbohydrate.

Most plant foods contain very little fat. However, modern food technology has made it possible to chemically remove these natural fats and process them into—oil! (Fourteen ears of corn—more than you could possibly eat at one sitting—are processed to make one tablespoon of corn oil containing 125 calories.) Adding these extracted and concentrated oils to the food we prepare or to the processed foods we buy greatly increases the caloric density of our diet. Look at what happens to a nutritious, low calorie potato:

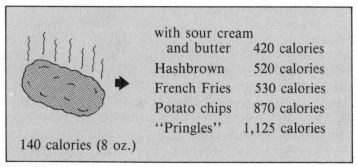

with sour cream and butter	420 calories
Hashbrown	520 calories
French Fries	530 calories
Potato chips	870 calories
"Pringles"	1,125 calories

140 calories (8 oz.)

FIG. 5.6:
Food Processing leads to Calorie Concentration

Our nutritious, low calorie potato has become a delivery system for fat. The price is also fattened: an 8-oz. potato sells for about fifteen cents; an eight-ounce can of Pringles sells for $1.49 "on special."

We don't mean to pick on Pringles. The same meteoric climb in calories and cost occurs when we convert a humble, nutritious apple into an out-of-this-world piece of pie a la mode: 75 calories rocket to 600! Or when we toast a piece of white bread to make it crisp and dry, add butter to make it soft and damp, and then add peanut butter and jelly to make it soar from 70 calories to 320. Or when we split a fresh, sweet banana, add fudge, nuts, ice cream and some gooey topping to make a 1000-calories nutritional disaster.

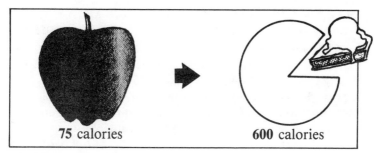

FIG. 5.7:
Food Processing Concentrates Calories

To show you how the addition of fats can easily turn a nutritious meal of only 685 calories into a caloric bomb of 1875 calories, take a look at Table 5.4.

Our food industry today is infinitely creative in condensing calories into all kinds of "snacks" for us to munch through-

Food	Cal.	Empty Calories	Cal.	Total Calories
Lettuce and Tomato Salad	40	+ Roquefort dressing	160	200
Whole Wheat Bread (1 slice)	65	+ Butter	70	135
Broccoli (½ cup)	35	+ Cream Cheese	130	165
Vegetarian Entree or Broiled Fish (6 oz.)	220	+ Tartar Sauce	80	300
Large Baked Potato with salsa	135	+ Hollandaise Sauce	180	315
Skim Milk (1 glass)	90	Whole Milk		160
Baked apple with date and walnut	100	Apple Pie a la mode (1/6)		600
Total Calories	**685**	**Total Calories**		**1,875**

TABLE 5.4:
Caloric Concentration: How fats do it!

out the day. We seldom wait till mealtime to eat. We "graze" habitually and continually. And we fatten like cattle.

ALCOHOL accounts for 9 percent of the calories adults consume every day. Two cans of beer carry 300 calories; two jiggers of 100 proof whiskey, 250; and two 3½ fluid ounce glasses of dessert wine carry 280 calories. And they, too, are purely empty calories. From the wine in our cooking to the beer at the ballgame, our current consumption of alcohol is at an all time high. Suprised? *Many people are when they realize that empty calories add up to 50 percent of all the calories we eat.* We are a society that is OVERFED and UNDERNOURISHED.

Please Don't Eat the Animals

Nearly everyone knows that Americans eat too much fat (and too little fiber). Around 40 to 45 percent of the calories we eat comes from fat (see Figure 5.4, page 42). About half of this amount comes from visible, or added fats and oils, as we've already discussed. The other half is not as readily seen because most of it is well hidden.

Hidden fats, the kind we often overlook, are almost all from animal products. In our "To Your Health" TV series, a man wearing a "Please Don't Eat the Animals" T-shirt helped explain where most of the fats are hidden: in meat,

Animal Product	Fat Content (% of total calories)
Steak	65-80%
Lamb	75%
Ham	80%
Bacon	85%
Hot Dog	85%
Whole Milk	50%
Cheeses	60-85%
Cream Cheese	90%

TABLE 5.5:
Fat Content (%) of Selected Animal Products
Because fat is well hidden, many people don't realize that meats and dairy products average from 50-85% of its calories as fat calories. Many "fake meats" or meat look-alikes are just as loaded with fat as the real McCoy.

Foods	% of total fat in US diet
Meats, Poultry & Fish	33%
Salad oils, Shortening, Lard	31%
Dairy Products	17%
Margarine & Butter	10%
Other	9%
	100%

TABLE 5.6: Source: *National Dairy Council*
Sources of Dietary Fat (US, 1985)
Of all the fat in the American diet, almost half of it comes from red meat and dairy products. It is well-hidden, and even more disturbingly, most of it is **saturated** fat.

cheese, cream, and milk.

Many people are surprised to learn that meat, especially *red meat, is the single largest source of fat in the U.S. diet.* While meat does supply many quality nutrients, it also provides an overabundance of fat calories and protein. Getting enough protein is not the problem. Actually, most Americans eat far too much protein. While many people eat 80 to 125 grams of protein each day, scientists have found that we need only 40 to 56 grams. Studies show that excess protein intake is actually harmful, contributing to kidney disease and osteoporosis. But even more serious is the heavy load of fat that most high protein foods carry.

Did you know that 50 percent of the calories in a glass of whole milk comes from fat, even though the carton says it contains only 3.5 percent fat? The "3.5 percent" is figured on the basis of weight, not calories. Since milk is largely

WHOLE MILK		3.5% fat by weight
Serving size		8 ounces
Calories per serving		160 calories
Fat per serving		9 gm
9 gm of fat x 9 cal/gm	=	81 calories
This means that 81 of the 160 calories in a serving of milk come from fat.		
81 ÷ 160 = .50 x 100 =		**50% calories from fat**

TABLE: 5.7:
How to Figure % of Fat (on the basis of total calories)

water, the fat-to-water ratio is quite low, but the fat-to-calories ratio actually is quite high.

If an 8-ounce package of cream cheese contains 850 calories and 86 grams of fat, you imagine the percent of fat in cream cheese? [86 grams x 9 calories per gram = 774 fat calories in a total of 850 calories = .9 x 100] = 90%!

Generally speaking, *animal products are very calorie-dense foods. They provide no fiber and very few carbohydrate calories, the body's preferred fuel. Instead they are loaded with fat and a lot of protein.*

How to Win the "Losing" Game

Mr. or Ms. Goodweight lives inside each one of us, but often stuck behind layers of laziness, bulges of self-indulgence, and mounds of misconceptions. Have you figured out how to find that slim and trim person inside yourself? That healthier you with the energy and self-confidence you used to have? Here are some keys to success:

Avoid refined and processed foods and eat less animal products. Instead, eat more food-as-grown, foods that are naturally low in calories and price and high in nutrition and fiber. These are high volume foods that will fill your stomach (your stomach can hold the equivalent of four cups of food) and give you the feeling of satiety. Once you reduce the concentrated calories and animal products in your diet, you can eat all the natural foods you want three times a day! You won't feel hungry and you'll lose one to two pounds a week consistently. It's a safe program that works—and it will keep you healthy.

Of course, some people still believe that starchy foods are fattening. They push aside their potatoes, rice and pasta (which carry about 4 calories per gram) and reach for the cheese and meat and other high fat foods (which carry 9 calories for every gram of fat they contain). Remember: the scientific way of winning the "losing" game is: *fats make fat, and unrefined starchy and natural foods make you slim!*

So forget about calorie counting, pills, shots, and the latest fad diet. Forget the rhythm method of girth control. Instead,

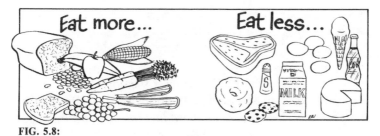

FIG. 5.8:
Dietary Key to Health and Weight Management:
Eat more unrefined plant foods. Eat less animal products and processed foods.
You can eat more volume, but your calorie intake is less!

get into a new lifestyle and stay with it: look for foods as
grown, such as whole grain breads and hot cereals (have
you tried a seven- or nine-grain cereal lately?), fresh fruits
(how about some papayas?) and vegetables (how about some
zucchini?). Help yourself to potatoes, yams and beans (there
must be over forty kinds). Pasta is perfect, and brown rice
is nice. Enjoy those baby carrots, cauliflowers, peas and
broccoli, the watercress and cherry tomatoes and try the 15
kinds of squash all in different colors! And season your food
with natural herbs (have you tried "Mrs. Dash," the low
salt, low pepper kind?) instead of oils, creams, and sauces.

When you make soups and hot cereal use your crockpot.
Put it to work while you sleep, knowing that your piping
hot, whole grain cereal will be ready when you wake up in
the morning: low in calories, loaded with good nutrition,
delicious and nutty in taste. And remember, meals made
with natural foods shouldn't take more than 15 to 25 minutes
to prepare, especially if you use your microwave oven and
waterless cookware efficiently.

Look at this as the beginning of a new lifestyle and an
end to all those crazy semi-starvation diets that left you
frustrated and unsatisfied, always craving more to eat.
Recondition yourself from old food preferrences and
patterns to new and better ways. A few short weeks spent
learning to prepare and enjoy delicious healthful food will
pay off for years to come. Shake your failure syndrome and
say "I can," because you can eat your way to better health,

you can have more energy, you can develop a better self-image, and you can cut your food budget in half (with the saving you can buy yourself a new wardrobe for that new body)!

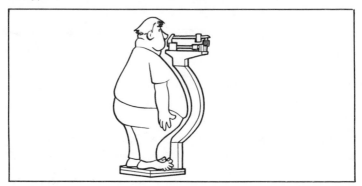

FIG. 5.9:
Focus on Health; don't focus on weight! Eat to live; don't eat to lose!

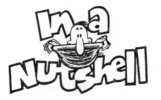

℞ How to Eat More and Weigh Less

1. *Let diets die!* Eat for health, and let the pounds take care of themselves.
2. *Eat more natural foods, simply prepared!*
   - freely use whole grain products, even pasta
   - freely use tubers and legumes, like potatoes, yams, squash, beans
   - freely use fresh fruits and vegetables (with low-calorie dressings)

- eat a substantial breakfast daily—a hot multi-grain breakfast will curb your appetite for hours, stabilize your blood sugar, emotions and nerves.
3. *Avoid refined, processed foods* and snacks high in fat and sugar.
4. *If you use animal products, use them sparingly,* more like a condiment!
5. *Drink plenty of water,* 6 to 8 glasses a day. Try herb teas, Perrier's, or just filtered water. Keep the sodas for special occasions.
6. *Walk briskly every day.* Begin with 5 to 10 minutes at a time and progress until you can do at least 30 minutes without fatigue.
7. *Picture yourself successful;* tie into supportive and spiritual resources. Remember: God didn't make a no-body. He created you for success. So, push on!
8. *Beware of weak moments:*
   - if one cookie leads to ten, don't eat the first one.
   - don't buy problem foods. If they are not around, you won't eat them.
   - if you are bored, frustrated, or lonely, don't snack; go for a walk, drink a glass of water, call a supportive friend, or "feast" on natural foods like semi-frozen grapes, melon or some juicy carrot sticks.
   - if you eat that "first" cookie, don't tell yourself, I've done it now, so I might as well eat the whole box! Instead, tell yourself, One cookie is not the end of the world, I'm going to stay with the program, I will lose weight as I keep at it!

6

Diabetes:
An American Special

What could be more American than baseball and Mom's apple pie? Here's what! Heart attacks! Strokes! Obesity! And another deadly disease: diabetes! A truly American special.

There are 30 million diabetics in the world. An estimated 16 million, or more than one half, are right here in this country. Nine million have been diagnosed, and an estimated seven million don't yet know they have the disease. A new diabetic is discovered every 50 seconds! And a newborn baby who lives to be seventy now has a 1-in-5 chance of becoming diabetic. The odds are getting worse.[1]

The disease and its vascular complications are responsible for 300,000 deaths a year, making diabetes one of the leading causes of death in the U.S.[2] Yet, surprisingly, this killer disease is virtually nonexistent in 80 percent of the world's population. Why? Because they can't afford it! They can't afford steaks and sodas, hamburgers and hot dogs, cheese and crackers, fries and pies. Societies less affluent than ours have substantially fewer diabetics because—are you ready— they eat better than we do!

Present Treatment: The Needle, the Pill, the Diet

In the TV series "To Your Health" we alluded to baseball statistics such as batting averages, games lost and won. What do you think of the following statistics?

Most diabetics are on the needle or on the pill. And all of them are supposed to be on some kind of a diet. Close to three million take insulin injections every day which control but don't cure. More than three million are on prescription drugs, drugs that seem to help, but that increase the likelihood of heart disease by 250 percent.[3, 4, 5] And another three million diabetics are on high protein diets, diets which increase the already serious risk of kidney disease.[6]

"Diabetes has been inexorably advancing, doubling every 15 years. Up to now there has been no known medical cure."

Diabetics spend an average of $600 a year each for medication and associated physicians' visits. The rest of us, through increased insurance premiums and tax dollars, paid in excess of $13 billion in additional health care services for diabetics last year.[7] And while the costs of diabetes are going up, many of the present therapies are proving frustrating and largely ineffective.

- Three out of ten diabetics end up in the hospital every year.
- Eight out of ten diabetics develop eye problems; diabetes is the leading cause of new blindness.
- Diabetics are eighteen times more likely to experience serious kidney damage than are nondiabetics; 25 percent of kidney dialysis patients are diabetics.[8]
- The Framingham Study has demonstrated that diabetes is a potent promoter of atherosclerosis.[9] Diabetes more than doubles the risk of heart disease and stroke. It can lead to sexual impotence, intermittent claudication, gangrene, (half of all foot and leg amputations in adults) and hearing impairment (see page 24).

Insulin injections, used since 1922, and oral diabetes drugs, introduced in the late 1950's, help to control the disease, but do not prevent or cure it. Up to now there's been no known medical cure.[10] Indeed, the problem is getting worse every year.

Since World War II, the incidence of diabetes has been inexorably advancing, especially among 45 to 54 year olds, at a rate of six percent per year, thus doubling every 15 years. Although some of this increase may reflect improvements in the detection of diabetes, the increase is real and troubling.

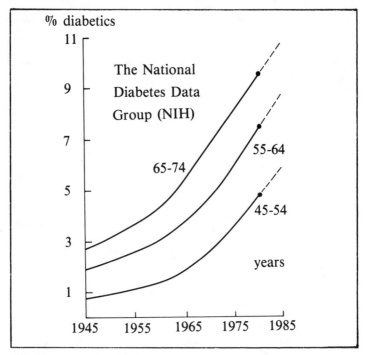

FIG. 6.1:
Trends in the Rate of Diabetes by Age Group (US 1945-1985)
The percentage of diabetics for selected age groups has steadily increased; i.e. the diabetes rate for those 45 to 54 years has gone from .8% in 1945 to 6% in 1985, an increase of more than 700%.

It is estimated that by 1990, ten percent or more of the population will fall victim to the disease.[11] Isn't it time to become disturbed? Shouldn't we search for a better game plan?

Just What *Is* Diabetes?

Diabetes occurs when the body becomes unable to handle glucose (sugar), and it piles up to dangerous levels in the blood. There are two different causes for this, and thus there are two different types of diabetes. **Type I Diabetes** afflicts 750,000 or 5 to 10 percent of all diabetics. In this type, the body doesn't produce any insulin at all. This disease is usually hereditary, although it can develop as a result of certain virus infections in which the insulin-producing cells of the pancreas are destroyed. The disease usually begins in childhood or youth and is commonly called "juvenile diabetes." Officially it is called "Insulin Dependent Diabetes Mellitus" (IDDM), because these people will always have to take insulin to survive; their lives depend on it. These diabetics are usually thin and rarely overweight.

Type II Diabetes is different. Commonly called "adult onset diabetes," and officially known as "Non-Insulin Dependent Diabetes Mellitus" (NIDDM), it afflicts an estimated 15 million Americans. This type usually hits after 40, as we get older and fatter, especially in the midsection. And most of these diabetics, when diagnosed, have *plenty* of insulin, but the insulin becomes blocked and cannot do its job properly.[12, 13]

What's *Really* Going On (in Type II Diabetes)?

Does diabetes come from the sugar bowl, eating too much sugar? Glucose, the body's form of sugar, does have an important role. The diabetic has too much glucose in the blood and urine and not enough in the cells. The cells need glucose, both for nourishment and to produce body energy. The problem revolves around insulin, a pancreatic hormone, a kind of chemical messenger, which enables glucose in the blood to enter into the cells.

When food is absorbed from the intestines into the blood, part of it is converted to glucose. Insulin then signals the cells to open their doors and take in the nourishment. If there is no insulin, or if the insulin is unable to perform its job, the cells cannot use the needed glucose. The cells starve while the glucose piles up in the blood, spills over into the urine and the person becomes—diabetic!

It's as though a grocery boy kept delivering bags of groceries on the person's doorstep but couldn't find the doorbell, or the bell was out of order. In the midst of plenty, the cells are famishing, and they are forced to look for another form of nourishment that can enter without the aid of insulin. Fat has the ability to do this. So the cells break down fats into fatty acids and use these to produce energy.

This process works, and is lifesaving, but it causes a great deal of havoc to the body. As glucose continues to build up in the blood, the filtering plant (kidneys) becomes overloaded, sugar spills into the urine and there is a good chance of a kidney strike. At the same time the breakdown of fat produces ketones, which in excessive amounts become poisonous to the body. The combination of excess glucose and ketones can cause fatigue, lethargy, confusion, coma, and sometimes death.

But why are the cells starving amidst plenty? What hinders the insulin from doing its vital and designated job? Why do people increasingly lose their ability to respond normally to their own insulin? Some answers have been coming in recently, and they relate to a better understanding of the concept of cell *receptors*.[14-16]

Cell receptors are the "door bells" that insulin must ring so that glucose can enter the cell. These are actual microscopic pits in the cell wall that are sensitive to insulin. In order to unlock the cell "door" to let the glucose in, insulin has to come in touch with these receptors. However, in most diabetics the cells are comparatively insensitive (resistant) to the action of insulin. The grocery boy comes to the door to bring needed cellular nourishment, but either the door bells (receptors) are not there, or the bells are resistant to the boy's touch—they don't work. In attempting

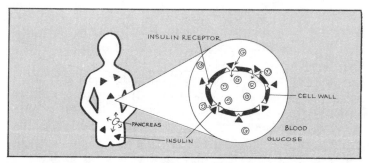

FIG. 6.2:
Normal Person   Rise in blood glucose G after a meal causes pancreas to produce insulin, which attaches to insulin receptors on cell surface, thus facilitating glucose entry and normalization of glucose in the blood.

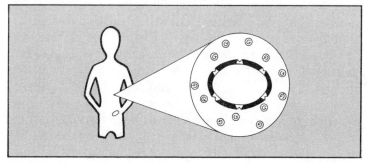

FIG. 6.3:
Type I Diabetic   Glucose cannot enter cell because pancreas cannot secrete insulin. Diabetic is *dependent* on insulin injections.

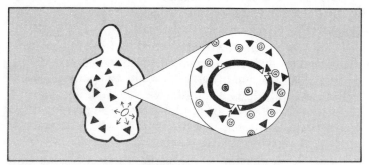

FIG. 6.4:
Type II Diabetic   Glucose cannot easily enter cell because hight fat levels and obesity interfere with function of receptors, thus opening fewer cells "doors." Glucose thus builds up in the blood instead of nourishing the cell.[38]

to cope with the increasing glucose levels, the pancreas produces more and more insulin. After years of overwork and abuse, however, the pancreas often suffers "burnout" and fails.

The problem in adult onset diabetes is usually not a defective pancreas, at least not initially, but a cellular insensitivity and resistance that relates to obesity and especially to a fat intake that in the American diet is typically excessive (we eat about three times more fat than the Japanese for instance.) Recent studies show excess fat intake can decrease the number of insulin receptors, and/or deactivate them.[17-19] This results in a gradual build up of glucose in the bloodstream. Conversely, a low fat, more natural diet (and the resultant weight loss) will not only increase the number of insulin receptors, but will cause them to become responsive to insulin once more.[20] The waiting glucose can then be accepted into the cell and used as it was meant to be.

A Self-Made Disease?

Type I (juvenile) diabetes is mostly hereditary, and from present knowledge those afflicted will need to take insulin for life—unless transplants of insulin producing cells become feasible.

But for the vast majority of diabetics it appears that their Type II diabetes is a disease of abundance that relates directly to the dramatic change in our American diet. What's the evidence?

J. Shirley Sweeney, M.D., showed as far back as 1927 that a high fat diet fed to healthy medical students produced a mild diabetic condition after only two days.[21] John Felber, M.D., in 1964 demonstrated that a similar high fat diet in nondiabetics raised insulin levels by 35 percent. This increased insulin level, however, was not high enough to prevent them from testing diabetic.[22]

James W. Anderson, M.D., professor of medicine and clinical nutrition at the University of Kentucky Medical College, evaluated the effect of diet composition on blood sugar levels. He was able to turn lean, healthy young men into mild diabetics in less than two weeks by feeding them a 65 percent fat diet, while a similar group, fed a 5 percent fat diet plus *one pound of sugar per day* did not produce even one diabetic after eleven weeks, when the experiment was terminated.[23]

Recently, Denis Burkitt, M.D., a renowned surgeon and medical researcher in England, cited the beautiful Pacific island of Nauru, where diabetes was unknown among the natives until a few years ago. They ate simply, mainly bananas and yams. But things changed. Nauru became a natural research laboratory when phosphates were discovered on the island. The natives suddenly became some of the wealthiest people in the world. The first thing they did, probably, was hire an all-American gourmet chef. Then they settled into a life of leisure, commerce and rich Western foods. The next thing they did was—develop diabetes. Thirty-five percent of the islanders over fifteen years of age now have the disease, highlighting the notion that adult onset diabetes is primarily a disease of dietary abundance, and not so much a disease of genetic make-up.

"Does diabetes come from the sugar bowl? Feeding one pound of sugar per day did not produce diabetes, but high fat intake will do it."

Aside from fat, fiber plays an important role in diabetes, not as a villain but as a hero.[24, 25] The fiber in plant foods absorbs water in the body, forming a natural "sponge." Food particles become suspended in this spongy mass, which allows them to be gradually absorbed into the bloodstream. This is nature's way of actually keeping the blood sugar on a more even keel, not allowing it to rise too rapidly. Sugared, refined and fiberless foods can cause a rapid rise in blood sugar levels, which trigger a swift pancreatic response: insulin is released to normalize the sudden glucose increase. But this response, under those circumstances, is sometimes "over-reactive," lowering the blood sugar to the point of producing symptoms of hypoglycemia. Natural fiber then prevents not only high upward swings in the blood sugar (diabetes), but it also prevents too rapid falls (reactive hypoglycemia).

In summary: The typically high fat diet combined with low fiber, middle age and obesity appears to set the stage for the development of adult onset diabetes.

Can Diabetes Be Prevented? Reversed? Cured?

As scientists have been uncovering the mechanisms that produce and promote adult onset diabetes, they are also discovering, or perhaps rediscovering ways to prevent it, reverse it, and perhaps even cure it.

In working with Nathan Pritikin at the Longevity Center in Santa Barbara, we found that a low fat, high fiber diet coupled with daily exercise enabled 26 of 32 diabetic patients (or 81 percent) to discontinue all oral diabetes drugs, and 11 of 22 diabetics (or 50 percent) to discontinue their daily insulin injections (the other 11 insulin-using diabetics had a substantial reduction in their insulin dosages). In less then four weeks on a low fat, high fiber diet coupled with daily exercise these diabetics, many of them with long-standing disease, were able to normalize their blood sugars without any medication.[26, 27] A follow-up study conducted two to three years later found sustained results, with most of the patients still free of oral drugs and insulin injections.[28]

The Pritikin studies were confirmed by the work of Dr. James Anderson,[29] one of the most respected authorities on diabetes in the world. When Kiehm and Anderson took thirteen diabetics off the 34 percent fat, 23 percent protein diet prescribed by the American Diabetes Association and fed them a 9 percent fat diet of mostly natural, high-fiber starchy foods, blood sugar levels were significantly lowered in all thirteen. All five patients taking oral drugs and four of the eight patients taking insulin were able to discontinue their medication completely.[30]

After working with low-fat, high-fiber, unrefined starchy food diets for fifteen years, Anderson stated: *"Ninety-five percent of adult onset diabetics on oral drugs could be off*

*such drugs in less than eight weeks, and 50 to 75 percent
could normalize their blood sugar and get off all insulin
within weeks.''* [31]

A fascinating recent study involved a group of Australian
aborigines who had left the Outback and moved to
Melbourne. As they adapted to their new lifestyle, many
developed diabetes, obesity and high blood pressure. They,
too, confirmed that diabetes can be an environmental
disease. But could it be reversed?

Dr. Kerin O'Dea of the University of Melbourne sent ten
middle-aged natives back to live and eat as they once had.
Their fat intake dropped from 40 percent to 13 percent of
total calories. They gave up their fatty, sugary diet of the
city and started eating once more natural foods found in
the Outback. As you might guess, their blood sugars
dropped significantly and their diabetes disappeared. And
it all happened in seven weeks![32]

It is fascinating and disturbing that *fat* has largely escaped
present-day incrimination as a major cause of diabetes,
considering the history of the disease in the last fifty years.

In the 30s fat was highly suspect. Israel Rabinowitch,
M.D., at the University of Montreal, reported his findings
from a five-year controlled experiment involving 100
diabetics on a 20 percent fat diet. Of his patients, 24 percent
were able to stop using insulin and return to normal
according to lab tests and clinical observation.[33, 34]

Then in 1935, Sir Harold Himsworth, M.D., at the
University Hospital in London showed in controlled
experiments that increasing the fat in the diet decreased a
patient's sensitivity to insulin so that more insulin had to
be injected. Himsworth established that the level of blood
sugar constantly changes in response to the amount of fat
in the diet.[35] However, by then insulin had been discovered
and its popularity pushed these early findings into the
background.

In 1955, Inder Singh, M.D., referring to Rabinowitch and
Himsworth, put 80 insulin-taking diabetics on an 11 percent

fat, natural foods diet. In less than six weeks, 50 of his patients were off insulin entirely, and after eighteen weeks all but twelve of his patients were off insulin injections. He wrote *"On a very low fat diet the endogenous insulin* (the insulin produced by the patient's own body) *begins to exert its curative effect within days, and most patients can be stabilized on such a diet plan alone, and some patients are totally cured."*[36]

He found that as long as patients tolerated the mild inconvenience of adjusting to a low-fat diet, their blood sugar levels did return to normal, and many could become free of diabetes. But his work was ignored, too.

But thanks to Pritikin, Anderson, O'Dea and others, we are back again—we hope finally—recognizing and rediscovering fat as the culprit it really is.

"Ninety-five percent of adult onset diabetics on oral drugs could be off such drugs in less than eight weeks, and 50 to 75 percent could normalize their blood sugar and get off insulin within weeks." —Prof. James Anderson, M.D.

Solutions and Recommendations

The "Baseball Diet"—the low fat, high fiber diet we talked about on TV—can help you win this deadly game. That's good news!

If you're a Type II (adult onset) diabetic, and almost all diabetics are, then chances are good that you can turn things around. *At least* 50 percent of the diabetics, even if they have taken insulin for years, can be off needles and pills in less than two months! The rest can substantially decrease their insulin dosage. And if you don't have diabetes, you can help make sure you don't ever get it. Here is the new game plan:

Highly refined sugary foods like cakes, candy and ice cream are part of the problem in that they contribute to obesity and can create an insulin "rush." A lack of fiber also plays a part. *But the main villain in diabetes is the enormous amount of fat in our diet.* Excess fat in the bloodstream strikes out the insulin receptors: the cells starve and the diabetic winds up in a slump. Kick the fats, grease and oils out of your diet. Instead, make a major trade: Fat, Oil and Sugar for Unrefined Food naturally high in fiber. These foods will help you beat diabetes. (And they can lower your cholesterol, helping you avoid the vascular complications of diabetes.)

"In the game of life, you are the coach. You are ultimately responsible for your health."

At this point in history, the Type II adult onset diabetic clearly has a choice: continued diabetes, insulin injections, oral drugs with their side effects, and continued dependence on the medical system—or, freedom from disease and drugs through the incorporation of a daily walking program and a healthy, simplified diet, which will also facilitate in weight control. Even Type I juvenile diabetics enjoy great benefits from this program. Their health improves, and their blood sugars are more stable with less insulin, and the ever-present threat of vascular complications is greatly reduced.

In the game of life, you are the coach. You are ultimately responsible for your health and for the health and well-being of your family. Make wise choices now that will maintain health and prevent diabetes, the American special.

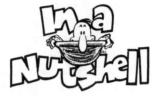

℞ How to Beat Diabetes (Type II)

Here is the "magic formula" that works (in most cases).

1. *Eat more natural fiber-rich foods, simply prepared, low in fats and grease and sugar.* Freely use whole grain products, tubers and legumes, salads and vegetables, and eat a substantial breakfast daily—a hot multi-grain cereal will curb your appetite for hours and stabilize your blood sugar.

2. *Use fresh whole fruits,* but not more than three servings/day.

3. *Avoid refined and processed foods* that are usually high in fat and sugar.

4. *Avoid fats, oils and grease.* If you use animal products, use them lean and very sparingly, more like a condiment. And watch oily and creamy dressings and sauces.

5. *Walk briskly daily.* Two 30-minute walks every day are ideal to help burn up the sugar in your blood.[37]

6. *Work with a physician* experienced in the effects of dietary therapy to monitor and adjust your drug needs.

Bibliography—Chapter 6

[1] National Diabetes Data Group, National Institutes of Health. (Personal communication.)

[2] Podolsky, S. (1978) (Guest Editor) Symposium on Diabetes. *Med Clin North America* 62:625-869

[3] Rifkin, H. (1978) Why control diabetes? in (Ed.) Podolsky S. *Med Clin North America* 62:747-752

[4] University Group Diabetes Program. (1970) *Diabetes,* Supplem. 2, 19

[5] part of the insert reads:
SPECIAL WARNING ON INCREASED RISK OF CARDIOVASCULAR MORTALITY: The administration of oral hypoglycemic drugs has been reported to be associated with increased cardiovascular mortality. This warning is based on the study conducted by the University Group Diabetes Program (UGDP), a long-term prospective clinical trial designed to evaluate the effectiveness of glucose-lowering drugs in preventing or delaying vascular complications in patients with Type II diabetes. The study involved 823 patients who were randomly assigned to one of four treatment groups. UGDP reported that patients treated 5 to 8 years with oral drugs had a rate of cardiovascular mortality approximately 2½ times that of patients treated with "placebo."

[6] West, KM. (1973) Diet Therapy of diabetes: an analysis of failure. *Ann Int Med* 79:425-434

[7] National Institutes of Health. (1985) Diabetes in America. NIH Pub. No. 85-1468

[8] *Ibid.*

[9] Garcia, MJ. et al (1974) Morbidity and Mortality in diabetes in the Framingham population. Diabetes 23:105-111

[10] Drury, TF, et al (1981) Prevalence and management of diabetes. *National Institutes of Health.* p. 25-31 (excerpt from position paper)

[11] Rushmore, CH. as quoted by Miles Robinson in *U.S. Senate Hearings* 99-513 on Nutrition and Physical Fitness in Public Health. (1986) US Gov. Printing Office, Washington, D.C. No. 58-1450

[12] Reaven, GM. et al. (1970) Study of the relationship between plasma insulin concentrations and efficiency of glucose uptake in normal and mildly diabetic subjects. *Diabetes* 19:571-578

[13] Berson, I. (1961) Plasma insulin in health and disease *Am J Med* 31:874-881

[14] Maugh, T. (1976) Hormone receptors: New clues to the cause of diabetes. *Science* 193:220-226

[15] Robinson, M. (1986) The Pritikin program and diabetes. *U. S. Senate Hearing* 99-513 on Nutrition and Physical Fitness in Public Health. US Gov Printing office, Washington, D.C. No. 58-1450:177-215

[16] Harvard Medical School Health Letter. (1985) The Diseases called "Sugar diabetes." Vol. 10:4, 1-4

[17] Davidson, P. (1965) Insulin Resistance in hyperglyceridemia. *Metabolism* 14:1059-1064

[18] Farquhar, J. (1966) Glucose, insulin, and triglyceride responses on high and low carbohydrate diets in man. *J Clin Invest* 45:1648-1653

[19] Olefsky, J. (1974) Reappraisal of the role of insulin in hypertriglyceridemia. *Am J Med* 57:551-556

[20] Buber, V. (1968) Improvement of oral glucose tolerance by acute drug induced lowering of plasma free fatty acids. *Schweiz Med Wsch* 98:711-712

[21] Sweeney, JS. (1927) Dietary factors that influence the dextrose tolerance test. *Arch Intern Med* 40:818-82

[22] Felber, JP and A Vannotti (1964) Effects of fat infusion on glucose tolerance and insulin plasma levels. *Med Exp* 10:1536-1541

[23] Anderson, JW. et al (1973) Effect of high glucose and high sucrose diets on glucose tolerance of normal men. *Amer J Clin Nutr* 26:600-607

[24] Philipson, H. (1983) Dietary fibre in the diabetic diet. *Acta Med Scand.* (Suppl.) 67:91-93

[25] McDougall, J. (1984) Food: the best medicine for diabetes and hypoglycemia. *Vegetarian Times.* Dec. 48-49

[26] Diehl, HA and D Mannerberg (1981) Regression of Hypertension, hyperlipidemia, angina and coronary heart disease in (Eds.) Trowell, HC and DP Burkitt. *Western Diseases: their emergence and prevention.* Arnold Publ. London 392-410

[27] Barnard, RJ. et al (1983) Longterm use of a high-complex-carbohydrate high-fiber diet and exercise in the treatment of NIDDM patients. *Diabetes Care* 6:268-273

[28] Barnard, RJ. et al (1982) Response of NIDDM patients to an intensive program of diet and exercise. *Diabetes Care* 5:370-376

[29] Anderson, JW. (1981) Regression of Diabetes in (Eds.) Trowell, HC and DP Burkitt. *Western Diseases: their emergence and prevention.* Arnold Publ. London. 373-391

[30] Kiehm, TG. et al. (1976) Beneficial effects of a high carbohydrate, high fiber diet on hyperglycemic men. *Am J Clin Nutr* 29:895-899

[31] Anderson, JW (1980) Diabetes: drugs or diet? (presentation) *Lifestyle Medicine Convention,* Loma Linda University, Loma Linda, CA

[32] O'Dea, K. (1985) (personal communication)

[33] Rabinowitch, IM (1931) Effects of low fat diet on diabetes and insulin. *N Eng J Med* 204:799-804

[34] Rabinowitch, IM (1935) Effects of the high carbohydrate low calorie diet upon carbohydrate tolerance in diabetes mellitus *Canad Med Assoc J* 33:136-144

[35] Himsworth, HP (1935) The dietetic factor determining the glucose tolerance and sensitivity to insulin of healthy men. *Clin Sci* 2:67-94

[36] Singh, I. (1955) Low-fat diet and therapeutic doses of insulin in diabetes mellitus. *Lancet I:*422-427

[37] Sornan, VR. et al (1979) *N Engl J Med* 301:1200-1204

[38] Liebman, B. (1982) Diabetes: foods, over pharmaceuticals *Nutrition Action* March:9-13

7

Hypertension: The Misunderstood Killer

Hypertension has nothing to do with nerves, although it is nerve-racking. It doesn't mean "hyper" or "tense." Hypertension is simply another word for High Blood Pressure and it can kill you.

Thirty-five million Americans have it. Another twenty-five million are "borderline"—living on the edge. People with high blood pressure are three times more likely to have a heart attack, five times more likely to develop heart failure, and eight times more likely to suffer a stroke than are people with normal blood pressure.[1]

Hypertension is **the** most important contributing factor in the 500,000 stroke cases reported every year, 150,000 of which do not survive. Forty percent of those who recover require special care for the rest of their lives; ten percent are permanently hospitalized. Approximately two million stroke victims in the United States are seriously limited because of paralysis—one of the crippling consequences of high blood pressure.[2]

Hypertension is also a very significant risk factor (remember the risk factor arch on page 28) in the 1,500,000 annual heart attacks. Together, strokes and heart attacks make cardiovascular disease the foremost cause of death, taking the life of every second American!

No one knows who among us will fall prey to hypertension. It can befall any age, creed or color, but it is common among people over 40. Fifty percent of the "over 40" age group, and seventy percent of those over 65, have it. And yet hypertension is uncommon in eighty percent of the world population.

We could do without it—we really could. And we are about to tell you how.

What It Is

It takes a certain amount of pressure to push two ounces of fresh, oxygenated blood per heartbeat through the 60,000 miles of blood vessels in your body. Each time your heart contracts (about once every second), blood pressure (BP) in your arteries increases. Each time your heart relaxes between contractions, the pressure decreases. So you have two blood pressure measurements: the "higher" (systolic BP) during contraction; and "lower" (diastolic BP) between contractions.*

When you are born, the walls of your arteries are flexible, elastic and muscular. They can easily handle the ebb and flow of normal blood pressure. Young children start the day with blood pressures of 80/40 or 90/50.** In many populations that youthful pressure seldom goes above 110/70—even in people who are over 70 themselves.

In our population, however, and in other industrialized societies, the so-called "normal" systolic blood pressure is often calculated as "100 + age"—i.e. 160 for a sixty-year-old. But this kind of "normal" blood pressure is *unhealthy* and high.

The National Institutes of Health define hypertension as any systolic pressure at or above 140 and any diastolic

---

* You can and should learn to take blood pressure readings. Ask your nurse or physician to show you how.

** Blood pressure is expressed in millimeters of mercury (mm Hg).

pressure at or above 90.[2] And every ten points above a systolic pressure of 140 increases the risk of heart disease or stroke by thirty percent. *Generally speaking, the lower your blood pressure, the better off you are.*

Occasional, transient increases in blood pressure are probably insignificant. But any **persistent high** blood pressure should be treated immediately, because this severe type of blood pressure can lead to irreversible damage of the kidneys, pancreas and retina of the eye. Hypertension, especially if it's associated with hardening of the arteries, can cause arterial "blowouts" in your brain or in your heart. It can leave you flat—on your back.

What Causes It?

Between five and ten percent of hypertension is caused by kidney disease, atherosclerosis in the kidney arteries, overactive adrenal glands, or adrenal gland tumors. But in at least ninety percent of the cases, the precise cause is obscure, and patients are said to have **essential** hypertension.

While we don't fully understand the exact cause of essential hypertension, there are four very definite and understandable contributing factors:

1. SALT

Lewis Dahl, M.D., of the Brookhaven National Laboratory discovered that a diet high in salt caused elevated blood pressure in laboratory animals.[3] Furthermore, through ingenious animal husbandry he was able to produce "salt sensitive" and "salt resistant" laboratory rats. The salt sensitive rats developed abnormally high blood pressures, while the salt resistant animals remained unaffected. He also observed that by increasing and decreasing the amount of salt, he could raise and lower the blood pressure of the salt sensitive animals.

Although most people aren't "rats," Dr. Dahl's work suggests that some people may be more susceptible to salt than others, and that "salt sensitive" people may be able to avoid hypertension by hiding the salt shaker.

Population studies of world health suggest that salt may be the Number One factor in hypertension. Many pre-industrialized peoples—the Australian aborigines, Greenland Eskimos, and tribes in New Guinea, the Solomon Islands, Africa, and Central and South America—consume very little salt, generally less than 0.5 grams per day.* These societies are characterized by a total absence of hypertension. In fact, their blood pressures often decrease with age.[4, 5]

It is salt, not the culture, that affects the blood pressure levels. Lot Page, M.D., found that the Lau tribe in the Solomon Islands, comparable to the other tribal groups in every other respect, did have considerably higher blood pressures. The apparent reason: the Lau traditionally boil their vegetables in sea water, thereby increasing their average salt intake to 15 to 20 grams per day.[6]

Compare the Lau tribe with farmers in northern Japan who preserve much of their food with salt and thus consume an average of 30 grams of salt per day. Sixty percent of these Japanese farmers have hypertension, and stroke is the most common cause of death.

In Africa Samburu farmers eat very little salt and have very little hypertension. However, when they're drafted into the army of Kenya their ration of salt goes up to 18 grams per day, and their share of hypertension increases proportionately.[7] Taken together, "without exception, low blood pressure societies are low salt societies. Not one person has high blood pressure, and a rise in blood pressure with age is rare," according to Lot Page, M.D.[8] And conversely, in societies where a lot of salt is used, mass hypertension follows mass salt consumption, just as migrants take on the diet and the blood pressure values of the host culture.

Once upon a time salt was scarce and high priced. Our historical regard for it shows in phrases like "salt of the earth" and "worth one's salt." Even the word "salary" is derived from the word "salt." But Americans consume too much of a good thing.

---

* 1 gm of salt = 1,000 mg of salt or 1/5 teaspoon of salt.

Salt is the second most used—and abused—food additive after sugar. Although salt (actually sodium chloride) is absolutely vital to life, we need only 500 milligrams (1/10 teaspoon) a day to stay in good health. By the time we are adults, most of us are consuming 15 to 20 grams (15,000 to 20,000 milligrams) of salt a day, twenty to forty times the amount we need. And about ten times more than our kidneys are designed to handle!

When you eat more salt than your kidneys are designed to cope with, excessive salt accumulates like a toxic waste that must be diluted before your body can handle it. So you begin to retain water, pounds of it, just to keep the salt diluted. At the same time your blood pressure goes up trying to shove all that extra salt water through the kidney filters.

To put it bluntly, if you're eating a typical American high salt diet, your kidneys are overworked and most of them will eventually lose the ability to function normally. You are on your way to high blood pressure.

Over the last three years a salt agreement has been reached among the scientific super powers. The Surgeon General, the Food and Drug Administration, the Department of Agriculture, the Department of Health and Human Services, the National Academy of Sciences and the American Heart Association have all urged the public to cut back on salt in order to reduce the risk and severity of hypertension and related diseases. *If we could cut our salt intake to 5 grams a day (one teaspoonful), we could solve one of our biggest health problems.*

James Charles Hunt, M.D., a leading hypertension specialist, has suggested that "with the reduction to no more than 5-grams of salt per day, hypertension could be prevented, and high blood pressure would probably disappear as a major public health problem."[9]

2. ARTERIAL PLAQUE

There is a war going on in us now. Plaque has infiltrated our blood supply lines, fat and cholesterol have become attached to the walls of our arteries and begun to harden. As the plaque builds up, restricting the free flow of blood through the arteries, our blood pressure goes up in trying to get food to the body. Blood pressure is always trying to help us, but if the "lines" get too narrow and the pressure gets too high, we could lose the war. Getting the excess fat and cholesterol out of our diets and our arteries would be a major step toward winning the war.

3. OBESITY

"The Battle of the Bulge" also directly contributes to high blood pressure. Fat has to be fed, too, and every pound of fat requires thousands of extra blood vessels. It takes higher blood pressures to get blood through them. Understandably, obese people are five times more likely to have hypertension.[10] Nearly everyone who is 20 percent or more overweight will eventually experience high blood pressure. It's just a matter of time. Many people have normalized their blood pressure by shedding excess weight.[11-13]

4. ESTROGEN

An added danger to women is estrogen, a hormone used in birth control pills and given to older women to control the effects of menopause. Estrogen is a salt retainer. It also increases the production of angiotension, a substance which raises blood pressure and reduces blood flow to the kidneys—a dangerous combination. The large 5-year Oral Contraceptive Study evaluating the effect of regular estrogen use on 46,000 women found an increase in cardiovascular mortality by up to 970 percent, depending on the duration of use.[14, 15]

"Three of the major four contributing factors of hypertension are diet-linked. We are committing suicide by the fork."

Did you notice that three of the four major contributing factos of high blood pressure are linked to our diet? We are committing suicide by the fork!

But high blood pressure can be stopped. It's not invincible.

As far back as 1948, William Kempner, M.D., at Duke University showed that with a severely restricted, almost sodium free diet, most hypertensive patients could normalize their blood pressure.[16] Then why haven't we wised up?

Ask those in the pharmaceutical industry. Several years ago they began making "wonder pills" that would de-salt the body. No more restrictive diets! A simple prescription, and people could eat whatever they wanted. The pills would take care of the problem. It was too good to be true.

Treating Hypertension: Procede With Caution!

Americans have a pet slogan, "If it ain't broke, don't fix it." Nearly all of us approach our health this way. We aren't concerned about maintaining it. We enjoy it, take chances on it, abuse it, seldom worrying about it—until something breaks down. Then we scramble for the "quick fix."

The quick fix for hypertension is a group of drugs called diuretics, or waterpills. Since the 50s, the diuretics have been the cornerstone of hypertension management. For years the most frequently prescribed diuretic thiazide drugs have been considered among the safest of the anti-hypertensive medications, and they are usually the first in a series of blood pressure medication to be given.

Diuretics force the kidneys to excrete abnormal amounts of salt and water. Once started, patients are usually told they *must take them for life.* "If you stop the pills," they are warned, "your blood pressure will go right back up." Other drugs are usually added, some to blunt the side effects, others to potentiate the effects of the diuretics.

Anti-hypertensive drugs do not cure high blood pressure, they only control it. If you stop taking them, your blood pressure races right back up again. And they cost a fortune, especially since you are supposed to take them for life. Of the nearly 20-million patients on these drugs, most take two or three different kinds to control their blood pressure. The average cost for medication and related visits to physicians is between $400 and $600 annually—per person. But money is not the only thing to be concerned about.

Significant international studies have recently shown that commonly prescribed diuretic drugs, like the thiazides, do indeed lower the risk for fatal and nonfatal strokes. However, they demonstrate *no such protection against coronary heart disease.* [17, 18]

Actually, some of these "blue ribbon" studies have shown a disturbing **excess** of coronary deaths. The large-scale government-funded Multiple Risk Factor Intervention Trial (MRFIT), a study costing more than $150 million, found that the coronary mortality was 70 percent *higher* in a group of hypertensive patients that received aggressive treatment when compared to a control group who received no treatment. [19, 20] The 5-year OSLO STUDY headed by Anders Helgeland, M.D., found that the incidence of sudden death among thiazide-treated patients was 300 percent (!) *higher* than of the control group who received no drugs. [21] And Gary Cutter, PhD., professor of biostatistics at the University of Alabama, found that the cardiac death rate (in a series of 5,000 angiographed patients) of those taking diuretics was 150 percent *higher* than the rate of those not taking these drugs.

Additionally, diuretic thiazides cause:

- consistent increase in blood *cholesterol* levels (by about 5 to 7 percent) promoting *atherosclerosis* [22, 23]
- increased *blood sugar* levels, promoting and aggravating *diabetes* [24, 25]
- increased *uric acid* levels leading to *gouty arthritis*
- depleted *potassium levels,* increasing the risk for *heart rhythm irregularities* and *sudden death* [26]

Considering the potential harm of thiazide diuretics, Dr. Freis recently challenged the concept of drug therapy for mildly hypertensive patients. In his editorial in the *New England Journal of Medicine* entitled, "Should Mild Hypertension be Treated?" he points out that treatment could be worse than the disease. [27] No wonder Norman Kaplan, M.D., a recognized authority in the field of hypertension treatment, warned, *"No single anti-hypertensive agent has more adverse effects than diuretic drugs. The benefits do not outweigh the risks, especially in older patients."* [28]

Aside from diuretics, other types of anti-hypertensive drugs, like Inderal, are commonly prescribed. Common side effects of these drugs include psychological depression, general lethargy, drowsiness and impotence.

Many people who take blood pressure pills for a while find their get-up-and-go just leaves without them. Their ambition goes, too; they miss the energy they once had; and often their sex life becomes a memory. Many of these patients believe these symptoms are a natural part of growing old. But they aren't, of course. *"Many physicians become so involved with the patient's blood pressure problem that they tend to be less aware of the quality of life aspects of the therapy,"* according to Dr. Sol Selvine, a Boston University behaviorist. [29]

"No single anti-hypertensive drug has more adverse effects than diuretic drugs."   Norman Kaplan, M.D.

It's no surprise that many people are less than enthusiastic about blood pressure pills. Despite major educational campaigns emphasizing the need for faithful and life-long drug therapy, as many as half of the patients stop taking anti-hypertensive drugs within a year and lose control of their blood pressure.

Still, taking pills—quick fixes—is easier than changing long-standing eating habits. Only seven percent of primary care physicians in Massachusetts felt they were "very successful" in helping patients to make dietary changes. In fact, only forty percent of the physicians felt that salt reduction was important for the average person. [30]

Even so, increasingly physicians and patients are beginning to take another look at nonpharmacologic approaches to treat mild hypertension. They are more interested than ever, especially since several recent studies have shown that a more comprehensive and educational lifestyle approach to this lifestyle problem can give excellent results.

What Can Be Done?

In a major study in California, 186 high blood pressure patients *(85 percent of the study group)* who had taken anti-hypertensive drugs for several years, were able to gradually reduce and finally *discontinue their medications after only four weeks.* Their average blood pressures came down to a normal 131/77. The dietary approach not only replaced their drug therapy, it produced lower blood pressures than the medication did, and there were no side effects to worry about.[31, 32] The patients were enthusiastic. At the end of one year, 82 percent were still off medication, and their blood pressures remained within normal limits.[33]

In another study researchers at the University of Mississippi Medical Center were able to demonstrate that 78 percent of hypertensive patients who had been on medication for at least five years were free of drugs and had normalized blood pressures after one year of using a low salt diet. Also those who were overweight lost each an average of ten pounds.[34]

"Major studies have shown that patients do not have to stay on drugs for life to control their blood pressure, if they change their diet."

Most hypertensive patients—all of them, really—would like to kick the drug habit. And most of them can, just by *reducing their excess weight and by reducing their salt intake to five grams a day.*

Salt, Salt Everywhere

Salt is ubiquitous in the American diet. An article in *Nutrition Action* recently noted that you can't get away from it even if you "brownbag a lunch consisting of a tuna salad sandwich on whole wheat bread, a strawberry yogurt and a glass of V-8 juice. These may not be bad nutritional choices for keeping your cholesterol and calories down and your vitamins and fiber up. But with regard to salt, you might as well have gone to the Golden Arches for a cheeseburger, because this nutritious alternative . . . packs over five grams of salt."[35]

McDonald's		"Brown Bag"	
Cheeseburger	2,000	Bran'nola Bread (2 sl.)	900
French Fries	250	Mayonnaise (1 Tsp.)	200
Vanilla Shake	500	Tuna (4 oz.)	1,300
Apple Pie	1,000	Strawberry Yogurt	505
		Campbell's V-8 (1 glass)	2,100
Total Salt (mg)	3,750	Total Salt (mg)	5,005

TABLE 7.1: Salt Content (in mg) in two meals

Though we all recognize that some foods are high in salt, like chips, pretzels and popcorn, amazing amounts of salt are hidden in processed foods. You may not recognize the salt because it's often masked by other flavors. In fact, most of us have eaten highly salted, sugared and peppered processed foods for so long and our taste buds have become so dulled that food critics have lamented the "death of the American palate." (See Table 7.2.)

Even processed foods we think of as sweet are salted. One cup of *Jell-O* chocolate pudding contains 1,200 mg of salt for instance, and every piece of coffee cake—any cake, for that matter—easily exceeds 1,000 mg.

Condiments, such as soy sauce, Teriyaki and Worcestershire sauces, catsup, mustard and bouillon cubes, are full of salt as listed in Table 7.3. Almost all commercially canned vegetables and soups are "salt mines."

There are myriads of invisible sources of salt, including food preservatives and flavor enhancers: monosodium glutamate (MSG), baking soda, sodium nitrate (curing agent for ham, bacon and hot dogs) and sodium benzoate.

Be careful about muffins, crackers, breads and ready-to-eat cereals. They account for 30 percent of the salt we eat.

Lunch meats, hot dogs, ham, sausages, bacon and even vegetarian meat substitutes are loaded with salt. Dairy products, especially pasteurized foods and brick cheeses, are extremely salty.

Natural foods are low in salt (actually sodium) and high in potassium, which help control blood pressure. But processed foods are low in potassium and skyhigh in salt.

TABLE 7.2: What Food Processing Does — Hidden Salt!

FOOD (Natural State)	SALT (mg)	FOOD (Com. processed)	SALT (mg)
Apple (1 fresh)	5	Apple Pie (1 slice)	500
White Beans (1 cup)	12	Canned Chili & Beans (1 cup)	3,000
Rice, brown (1 cup)	12	Minute Rice (1 cup)	1,000
Wheat Flakes (2 oz.)	20	Wheaties (2 oz.)	1,850
Potato (1 fresh, 5 oz.)	20	Frozen Pasta au gratin (1 cup)	2.750
		Potato Chips (5 oz. bag	3,500
Tomato (1 fresh)	35	Tomato Sauce (½ cup)	1,950
		Canned Tomato Soup (1 cup)	2,200
Beef, lean	140	Corned Beef	2,360
Milk (1 cup)	300	Cheese, American (2 slices)	2,050
Chicken (8 oz.)	300	Kentucky Fried Chicken (3-piece dinner)	5,600

"Seventy-five percent of the salt eaten is in processed food, 10% occurs naturally in food, and 15% comes from the salt shaker."

TABLE 7:3: Salt and Condiments (SALT "BOMBS")

CONDIMENT	Amount	SALT (mg)
Ketchup	3 tsp.	1,100
Italian Dressing	3 tsp.	2,500
Soy sauce	1 tsp.	2,500
Dill pickle	1 large	3,000
Garlic salt	1 tsp.	4,500
Salt	1 tsp.	5,000

It is this combination of processed and fast foods that account for 75 percent of our salt intake. (See Table 7.2.) Only ten percent comes from unrefined, natural foods where salt resides as sodium. The rest comes from the salt shaker, either at the dinner table or during cooking.[35]

While manufacturers are not required to list the salt content of their products, a quick glance at the label will tell you a lot. Watch for words like "salt," "sodium" and "soda" on the label, and notice their position on the list of ingredients. As a rule of thumb avoid products where "salt" terms appear among the first five ingredients.

Also be aware of the new packaging terminology proposed by the FDA:*

"Sodium-free"	5 mg or less
"Very low Sodium"	35 mg or less
"Low Sodium"	140 mg or less
"Reduced Sodium"	a 75 percent decrease

The Salt Solution

When Ronald Reagan was governor of California, a physician told him he could live fifteen years longer** "if he stopped salting his food." "In less than a week, I cured myself of the salt habit," the President said. (Some barbs have suggested it's the one "Salt agreement" he's been willing to live with!)

The President is an excellent example of how diet can help keep you in your prime. We jokingly call it the *"100-Year-Old Diet"*—but there's no reason why you shouldn't expect to be around and healthy at 100. Keeping or getting your blood pressure normal will help.

Here are some guidelines to "shake the habit":

1. Avoid high salt foods
- Avoid fast foods wherever possible, as well as salted snacks.

---

* Sodium Chloride, common table salt, is 40% sodium. To convert sodium to salt, multiply the amount of sodium by 2.5. To convert salt to sodium, multiply the amount of salt by .4.

**Metropolitan Life statistics predict that the life expectancy for a 35-year-old man is reduced by 15 years, if the BP is greater than 150/100 mm Hg.

- Avoid processed foods such as hot dogs, lunch meats, pasteurized cheeses, canned vegetables and soups, frozen dinners and commercially prepared entrees, instant and ready to eat cereals.
- Avoid commercially baked goods, including cakes, pies, cookies and some breads, unless they're low in salt.
- Avoid foods preserved in brine, such as corned beef, sauerkraut, ham, pickles, olives and sardines.
- Avoid condiments high in salt, such as soy sauce, MSG, garlic and onion salt (the powder is okay), and salad dressings, unless they are low in salt and fat.

2. Ban the salt shaker from the table, or buy one with one-third the number of holes in the top, or put the salt in the pepper shaker. Do not salt food while cooking. Instead learn to season with fragrant herbs and zesty spices. There are several tasty salt-free or low-salt seasonings available at the supermarket. Look for *New Vegit, Health Valley* or the salt-free *Mrs. Dash* label.

3. Read labels when you're shopping. You'll find now all kinds of new *low* sodium products.

4. Eat an abundance of unrefined foods, which are naturally low in sodium, and season with herbs. Just eating foods closer to their natural state will reduce blood pressure by about ten percent,[36] and will facilitate weight loss, a pound or two a week. Fresh fruits and vegetables are high in potassium, which will contribute to a more favorable potassium-sodium ratio and help in blood pressure normalization.

5. When eating out, order food as *you* would like it cooked, not as they want to cook it. After all, you're the one who's paying for it.

Nearly every restaurant includes a "cooked cereal" (or Shredded Wheat) and "fresh fruit in season" on its breakfast menu. Stewed prunes and applesauce is usually available also. Add whole wheat toast, slice a banana on top and you're off to a good start. Just pass up the bacon and eggs, of course.

At salad bars, fill your plate with greens and chopped vegetables. Avoid croutons, bacon bits and foods that are pickled, marinated or in creamy dressings. Ask for lemon juice, or low-salt, low-fat dressings, or bring your own.

Baked potatoes and cooked vegetables are nearly always available. Ask for these to be served without toppings, butter or salt. Plain yogurt, chives, cottage cheese, fresh dill, sliced tomatoes or a salsa make excellent toppings.

6. Be a good sport and be patient. Your taste buds will adjust. Initially, people on a low salt, more natural diet complain that their food tastes flat and bland. After two to three weeks—most people actually survive!—it tastes *better*. Remember that taste is not so much determined by your oral cavity as by what happens above the ear lobes. The salt-loving palate is a learned attitude. You can change that. Should somebody try to "salt-poison" you with a commercially prepared soup after having been on a low salt diet for a couple of weeks, watch out: you'll wonder how you could have ever enjoyed such briny solutions.

The Natural Solution

Some of the answers to the misunderstood killer are found in

(1) SALT REDUCTION—REPLACE WITH HERBS!

(2) WEIGHT REDUCTION

When weight is reduced, blood pressure usually falls. Studies have shown that for every two pounds of excess weight lost, the systolic BP drops 1 to 1.5 points.[11-13] (This drop occurs independent of salt reduction.)

(3) FAT REDUCTION

Carefully controlled and sophisticated experiments have demonstrated that cutting the average US fat intake in half will lower the blood pressure by about 10 percent while keeping weight and salt intake constant.[36] It is thought that the reduction in blood viscosity, which results from eating less fat, produces these favorable blood pressure changes.[32, 37, 38]

(4) PHYSICAL EXERCISE

Although the direct effect of daily exercise on blood pressure is not quite clear yet, a regular walking program facilitates weight control, helps to dissipate tension and stress and improves circulation and well-being.

With a lifestyle program like this, there is no reason that we shouldn't enjoy bouyant health, sharp minds and live a full 100 years.

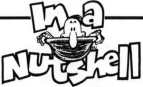

℞ How to Lower Your Blood Pressure

1. *Substantially lower salt intake*
2. *Avoid processed and fast foods* high in fat and salt
3. *Avoid empty calories* such as fats, oils and sugar
4. *If you eat animal products like cheese and meat, learn to use them sparingly*
5. *Lose excess weight*
6. *Eat plenty of natural foods,* simply prepared, low in fats and salt, but usually high in potassium. Freely use whole grain products, potatoes and legumes, salads and vegetables, and don't forget the fruits!
7. *Walk briskly daily.* Progress to 30 to 60 minutes daily.
8. *If you are using blood pressure medication,* ask your doctor to help you incorporate diet therapy and appropriate lifestyle changes into your program. Your doctor can give you careful supervision in adjusting your drug dosages—as you eat and exercise your way out of hypertension.

Bibliography—Chapter 7

[1] Kannel, WB et al. (1984) Optimal resources for primary prevention of atherosclerotic diseases: Atherosclerosis Study Group. *Circulation* 70:153A-205A

[2] Subcommittee on Definition and Prevalence of the 1984 Joint National Committee. (1985) Hypertension prevalence and the status of awareness, treatment, and control in the United States. *Hypertension* 7:457-458

[3] Dahl, LK (1960) Possible role of salt intake in the development of essential hypertension in (Eds.) Reubi, Bock, Cottier. *Essential Hypertension* (Springer, Berlin) pp. 53-65

[4] Blackburn, H. and R. Prineas (1983) Diet and hypertension: anthropology, epidemiolody, and public health implications. in (Ed.) Hegyeli, RJ. *Nutrition and cardiovascular disease.* (Karger, Basel) pp. 31-79

[5] Gleibermann, L (1973) Bloodpressure and dietary salt in human populations. *Ecology of Food and Nutr.* 2:143-156

[6] Page, LB et al. (1974) Antecedents of cardiovascular disease in six Solomon Island societies. *Circulation* 29:1132-1146

[7] Shaper, AG et al. (1969) Bloodpressure and body build in three nomadic tribes in Northern Kenya. *E Afr Med J* 46:273-281

[8] Medical News (1977) More proof of salt-hypertension link. An interview with Lot Page. *JAMA* 237:1305-1308

[9] Hunt, JC (1977) Management and treatment of essential hypertension in (Eds.) Genest J, Koin E and O. Kuchel. *Hypertension* (McGraw-Hill, NY) pp. 1068-1117

[10] Kannel, WB et al. (1967) Relation of adiposity to blood pressure and development of hypertension: the Framingham Study. *Ann Intern Med* 67:48-59

[11] Reisin E et al (1983) Cardiovascular changes after weight reduction in obesity hypertension. *Ann Intern Med* 98:315-319

[12] Reisin E et al. (1978) Effect of weight loss without salt restriction on the reduction of blood pressure in overweight hypertensive patients. *N Engl J Med* 298:1-6

[13] Maxwell, MN et al. (1984) Bloodpressure changes in obese hypertensive subjects during rapid weight loss: comparison of restricted vs. unchanged salt intake. *Arch Intern Med* 144:1581-1584

[14] Royal College of General Practitioners (1981) Oral Contraceptive Study. *Lancet* 1:541-548

[15] Fisch, IR and J Frank (1977) Oral Contraceptives and bloodpressure. *JAMA* 237:2499-2503

[16] Kempner, W (1948) Treatment of hypertensive vascular disease with rice diet. *Am J Med* 4:545-577

[17] Medical Research Council (1985) MRC trial of treatment of mild hypertension: principal results. *Br Med J* 291:97-104

[18] Whelton, PK (1983) New trial tightens link between thiazides and cardiac arrhythmia. *Med World News* 32:Jan.24

[19] MRFIT: Risk factor changes and mortality results (1982) *JAMA* 248:1465-1477

[20] Kuller, LH et al. (1980) Primary prevention of heart attacks: MRFIT. *Am J Epidemiol* 112:185-191

[21] Helgeland, A. (1980) Treatment of mild hypertension, a 5-year controlled drug trial. The Oslo Study. *Am J Med* 69:725-732

[22] Grimm, RH (1981) Effects of thiazide diuretics on plasma lipids and lipoproteins in mildly hypertensive patients. *Ann Intern Med* 94:7-11

[23] Goldman, AI et al. (1980) Serum lipoprotein levels during chlorthalidone therapy. *JAMA* 244:1691-1696

[24] Ames, RP and P Hill. (1982) Improvement of glucose tolerance and lowering of glycohemoglobin and serum lipid concentration after discontinuation of antihypertensive drug therapy. *Circulation* 65:899-904

[25] Murphy, MC et al (1982) glucose intolerance in hypertensive patients treated with diuretics; a fourteen-year follow-up. *Lancet* 2:1293-1294

[26] Holland, OB (1981) Diuretic induced ventricular ectopic activity. *Am J Med* 70:762-768

[27] Freis, ED (1982) Should mild hypertension be treated? (editorial) *N Engl J Med* 307:306-309

[28] Kaplan, N. (1985) Diuretics: where shall we go from here? *Hospital Tribune.* May 16

[29] Selvine, S (1986) quoted in *Los Angeles Times* Study warns of hypertension medicines' side effects. June 26

[30] Wechsler, H et al (1983) The physician's role in health promotion—a survey of primary-care practitioners. *N Engl J Med* 308:97-100

[31] Diehl, HA and D Mannerberg. (1981) Regression of hypertension in (Eds) Trowell HC and DP Burkitt. *Western Diseases: their emergence and prevention.* (Arnold Publ., London) 392-410

[32] Barnard, RJ et al (1983) Effects of a high complex-carbohydrate diet and daily walking on blood pressure and medication status of hypertensive patients. *J Cardiac Rehabil* 3:839-846

[33] Diehl, HA and D Abbey (1981) 1-year follow-up on 186 formerly hypertensive patients. Loma Linda University, unpublished

[34] Langford HG et al (1985) Dietary therapy slows the return of hypertension after stopping prolonged medication. *JAMA* 253:657-664

[35] Jacobsen, M et al (1983) Salt, salt everywhere. *Nutrition Action* Nov. pp 6-9

[36] Puska P, Iacono JM et al (1983) Controlled, randomised trial of the effect of dietary fat on blood pressure. *Lancet* 1:1-5

[37] Iacono, JM et al (1982) The role of dietary essential fatty acids and prostaglandins in reducing blood pressure. *Prog Lipid Res* 20:349-364

[38] Barnard, RJ et al (1985) Effects of diet and exercise on blood pressure and viscosity in hypertensive patients. *J Cardiac Rehabil* 5:185-190

8

Cholesterol: The King Pin

What can turn a healthful, normal and needed substance into a dangerous killer? How can something that helps building bones, making sex hormones and balances the body's stress response also choke off needed oxygen and damage vital organs and tissues?

Cholesterol—is both the hero and the villain. While we cannot live without it, in excessive amounts it becomes a serious threat, and often an outright killer.

The cholesterol level is the single most important factor in determining one's risk of developing cardiovascular disease. The famous Framingham Study and the recently published MRFIT study have clearly shown that a person with a blood cholesterol level of 260 mg% is *four times* more likely to have a fatal heart attack than is a person with 200 mg% or less.[1] In other words, an increase of 60 points in one's blood cholesterol level increases the risk of dying of heart disease by *400 percent!* This does not mean that a blood cholesterol level of 200 mg% is healthy. It is *not*.

The Case Against Cholesterol

The International Atherosclerosis Project studied autopsied arteries from all over the world, searching for evidence of arterial damage and plaque.[2] Coronary and brain arteries from deceased people in fourteen countries were carefully examined, some 23,000 arteries in all. The overwhelming evidence proved that:

1. The degree of atherosclerosis (plaque build up in the arteries) is directly proportional to the frequency of coronary heart disease and stroke, and cannot be explained as part of the aging process.

2. Cholesterol and fat levels in the blood are directly related to plaque damage.

Angiograms of the coronary arteries were done on 723 men under the age of forty who were admitted to the Cleveland Clinic with slight chest pains.[3] These X-ray pictures showed that the extent of arterial closure was directly related to their blood cholesterol levels. Twenty percent of the men who had 200 mg% blood cholesterol had significant (50 % or more) arterial closure; sixty percent of those with 251-275 mg% cholesterol—and *ninety-one percent* of those with 350 mg% and above—had significant arterial closure (see Fig. 8.1).

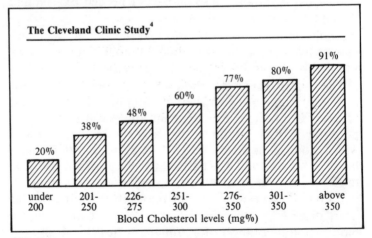

The Cleveland Clinic Study[4]

FIG. 8.1:
Blood Cholesterol and Serious Coronary Artery Disease. The higher the cholesterol level, the higher the incidence of significant artery narrowing. So-called "normal" US cholesterol levels are "deadly."

The results of the Cleveland Study were clear: blood cholesterol level is the most reliable predictor of arterial closure—in any age group.[4]

In another major study, Ancel Keys, Ph.D., and his team observed more than 12,000 men in seven different countries over a period of twelve years.[5] This study found clear connections between heart disease and blood cholesterol.

For instance, during this period there were fourteen times as many fatal heart attacks in Finland as there were in Japan. While the Finns' average cholesterol level was 264 mg%,

---

"Eighty-seven percent of all coronary deaths could be prevented, if the cholesterol was kept below 182 mg%, blood pressure was under 120, no smoking or diabetes." [41]
Prof. J. Stamler, M.D.

---

the Japanese men averaged 140 mg%. The cholesterol level in both groups was strongly affected by the amount of saturated fats—from animal products—found in their diets.

Further research showed that when Japanese men migrated to California, they left behind their low fat, low cholesterol diet—and their apparent immunity to heart disease.[6] Their fat intake moved from 10 percent to 40 percent of total calories, their blood cholesterol went up from an average of 150 to 228 mg%, and their death rate due to coronary disease increased tenfold, almost equal to the death rate of American males.

Two hundred such migrant studies confirm that atherosclerosis is not so much a disease of genetics as it is a disease of lifestyle. As "protected" people move to a coronary-prone culture with its dietary excesses, they quickly begin to develop the diseases of the host country.

Even though the Japanese smoke more and have higher blood pressures than we do, there is very little atherosclerosis in Japan. Not too long ago it was so rare that Japanese medical schools had to import plaque-filled coronary arteries from Johns Hopkins University in Baltimore to demonstrate to their medical students the disease that was killing every other American!

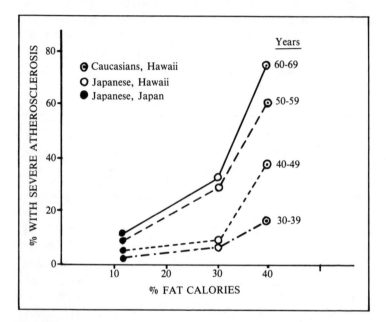

FIG. 8.2:
Fat Intake Levels and Extent of Atherosclerosis.[6] International autopsy studies show that as people eat more fat and cholesterol, the extent of arterial plaque increases. Japanese on a very low fat diet have minimal atherosclerosis, which changes, however, as they adopt higher fat and animal diets. In fact, Japanese men living in the US had more artery damage at 30-39 years, than those living in Japan had by the age of 70(!)

Jeremiah Stamler, M.D., at Northwestern University School of Medicine indicted our rich diet, reflected in our elevated cholesterol levels, as the *"primary, essential* and *necessary* cause of the current epidemic of atherosclerotic disease in Western industrialized countries. Cigarette smoking and hypertension are only secondary or complementary causes."[7]

For at least a decade it has been generally known that blood cholesterol levels below 160 mg% protect populations from atherosclerosis. Antonio Gotto, M.D., president of the American Heart Association, stated in a U.S. Senate hearing that "In societies where the blood cholesterol is under 160 mg% there is virtually no coronary artery disease or atherosclerosis."[8] His conclusion?—"If we lower the cholesterol count of everyone in the United States to below 150 mg%, we would probably wipe out heart disease."[9]

Dr. William Castelli of Framingham fame went a step further, saying that "Diet could *reverse* coronary artery disease in ninety percent of patients if we could get everybody's cholesterol below 150 mg%." [10]

The ideal blood cholesterol level is 100 plus age, not to exceed 160 mg%.* Anything above 160 mg% carries risks. [13, 40, 41]

Risk	Blood levels (mg%) for	
	cholesterol	LDL cholesterol
IDEAL	100 plus age*	less than 90
ELEVATED	161-180	90-110
HIGH	181-220	111-150
VERY HIGH	221-260	151-190
DANGEROUS	above 260	above 190

TABLE 8.1:
Risk of Coronary Heart Disease and Cholesterol Levels.

Recently much discussion has focused on high levels of HDL cholesterol (the "good" cholesterol) and on HDL/LDL ratios.[12] Since HDL can be influenced by alcohol, estrogen use, pesticides, etc., and since the HDL adds considerable cost to an otherwise inexpensive blood test, we consider blood cholesterol as probably the best determinant of early coronary heart disease.

---

* Plaque regression (gradual shrinking) usually begins at "ideal" cholesterol level, reducing the need for coronary bypass surgery.[11, 35]

"Normal" vs. "Ideal" Cholesterol Levels

Extensive research over the past two decades has clearly shown that cholesterol levels of 300 and up are lethal, levels of 210 (the American average) are dangerous and levels of 160 and below are desirable. The incidence of cardiovascular disease in population groups with blood cholesterol levels of 70-140 mg% is extremely rare, with 140-180 mg% it is less rare, but it becomes epidemic in groups with blood cholesterol levels over 180 mg%.

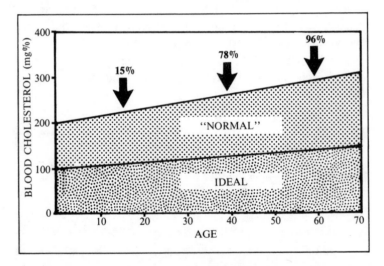

FIG. 8.3:
Probability (in %) of significant arterial narrowing according to age and cholesterol.

Irving S. Wright, M.D., in an editorial in the Journal of the American Medical Association concluded that accepting the current average cholesterol readings as normal is "both confusing to many physicians and detrimental to the proper care of patients. The physician who accepts such laboratory 'normals' is not acting on the basis of the best scientific criteria, and his patient may be misguided in planning his dietary pattern."[13]

Unfortunately and dangerously, for years we have accepted cholesterol levels of 150-300 mg% as "normal" in our society because ninety percent of Americans fall into that range. While these values may be common for Americans, they certainly are not healthy. Instead, they are norms for a society where every second person dies of atherosclerosis. There is no consolation in being "normal" concerning one's blood cholesterol. Such levels are often passports to disability and death. "Ideal" levels are what we want.

How Plaque Develops

More than a hundred years ago a German pathologist, Rudolf Virchow, M.D., discovered the cholesterol-atherosclerosis connection. He examined plaque, a kind of arterial "rust" taken from diseased arteries, and found that it consisted of a fibrous, wax-like substance which turned out to be mostly cholesterol. He theorized that an injury to the endothelium, the thin, innermost lining of the artery, caused plaque to form.

Many researchers now believe that atherosclerosis is indeed related to this process. First, the sensitive endothelial cells lining the artery must be damaged, either mechanically or biochemically, and secondly, elevated fat and cholesterol circulating in the blood must be present allowing excess fat and cholesterol in the blood to leak into the muscle layer of the artery. This irritates the muscle cells which then engulf the cholesterol and multiply, eventually forming a bulge inside the artery which restricts and ultimately obstructs the flow of blood.[14, 15, 51]

But what causes the damage? Oxygen starvation—that's the problem! With a shortage of oxygen in the blood, the endothelial layer becomes **biochemically** altered. The permeability changes. The lining becomes "porous" permitting fats and cholesterol to enter the muscle layer setting up an inflammatory process.[16]

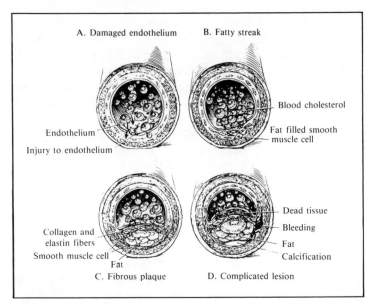

FIG. 8.4:
Progressive Steps in Plaque Formation.

A. Once the endothelium has been injured, toxic substances like cholesterol (LDL) may enter the arterial wall.
B. Special muscle cells within the intima become filled with fats forming a fatty streak.
C. A fibrous plaque develops containing cholesterol, collagen and calcium.
D. A complicated lesion builds up that extends into the inner lumen of the artery, eventually leading to "suffocation" of target organs.

If the blood cholesterol is 160 mg% or less, the endothelial injury will usually heal and the bulge will shrink. However, with typical American cholesterol levels over 200 mg%, fat and cholesterol particles continue to leak through the endothelial layer into the muscle layer and further aggravate the inflammatory process. The result is the formation of fibrous scar tissue that hardens into "plaque."

Plaques are like tire patches: they are the body's response to damage to the arterial wall. Tragically, in responding to the continued irritation over the years, the plaque gradually

"If you want to lose weight, eat like a horse!" THE HORSE DIET

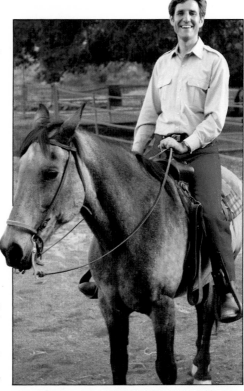

Dr. Diehl is showing Pastor Tucker the brain, "the incredible magic of ultimate design."

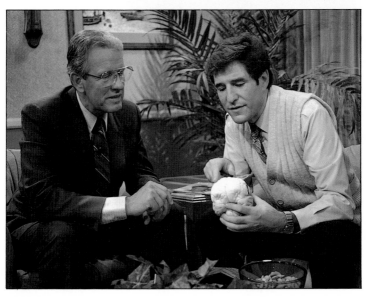

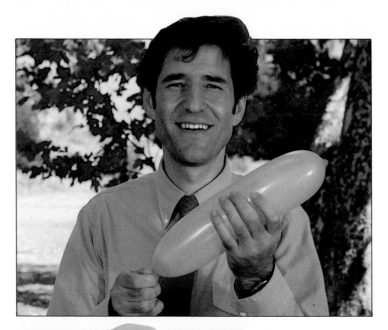

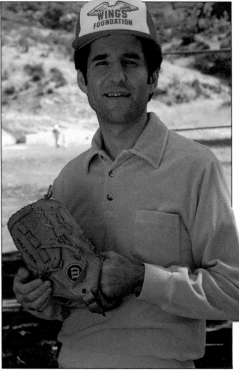

▲
"As a child, your
arteries were flexible
like a balloon."
**THE 100-YEAR-OLD
DIET**

"To win against
diabetes, we need a
new gameplan."
**THE BASEBALL
DIET**
◄

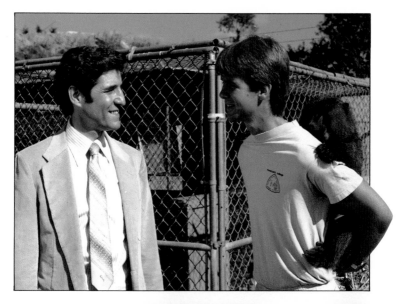

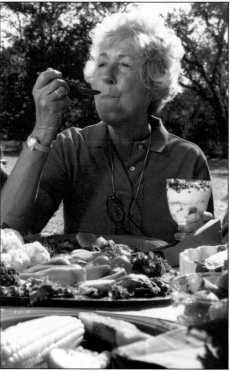

"Monkeys normally don't die of heart attacks."
THE MONKEY DIET

"Eat yourself healthy!"
THE OPTIMAL DIET
▶

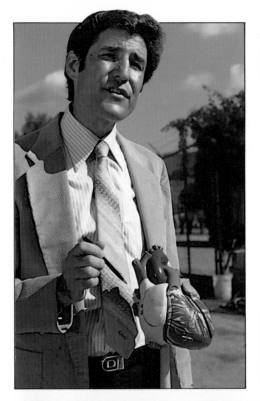

"Hearts shouldn't attack *us*, and they wouldn't if we ate differently."

Pastor Tucker and Dr. Diehl on the Search television set at The Quiet Hour recording studios.

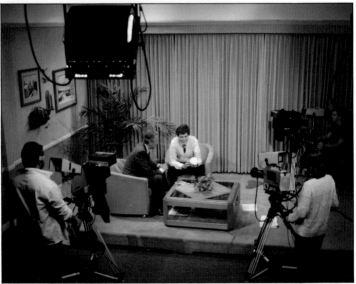

enlarges until it eventually interferes with bloodflow, or obstructs it entirely.

And what causes insufficient oxygen supply in the blood?

1. **Smoking can do it.** Red blood cells work day and night picking up and carrying oxygen to the cells of the body. However, when carbon monoxide—a constituent of cigarette smoke—is inhaled, it enters the bloodstream and attaches (with an affinity that is 200 times stronger than that of oxygen) to the red blood cells, which are then unable to carry their share of oxygen. The result: the oxygen level in the bloodstream is lowered. That's one of the major reasons why smokers, especially those on high fat, high cholesterol diets, have a 250 percent greater death rate from heart disease than do non-smokers.

2. **Diet can do it.** Fats in the blood reduce the oxygen supply in two ways: by slowing circulation and by reducing the oxygen carrying capacity of the red blood cells.[17] When fat enters the bloodstream it acts as an adhesive surrounding these cells, causing them to cling together. These clumps of red blood cells can no longer pass through some of the body's microscopic capillaries. As much as 20 percent of the capillary capacity can be thus blocked, slowing circulation, and producing oxygen starvation in many of the tissues.[18] The clumps not only block the capillaries, but are

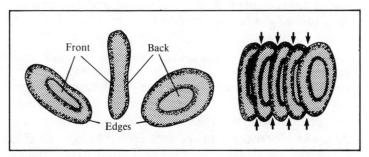

FIG. 8.5:
Design of Red Blood Cell (RBC) maximizes surface area and minimizes volume. Oxygen is carried on the RBC surfaces, which become greatly reduced when RBC's clump in response to high fat diet.

unable to deliver their normal load of oxygen. Single file, each red blood cell carries useable oxygen over its entire surface, but if the cells are bunched, only the outside surface of the bunch can deliver oxygen to the vessel walls.

To illustrate how a high fat meal can interfere with proper oxygenation and create angina pain, Peter Kuo, M.D., at the University of Pennsylvania, after an overnight fast, gave each of fourteen angina patients a glass of heavy cream and measured the fat increase in their blood.[19] Six of the patients experienced chest pain identical to the pain they experienced climbing stairs. Dr. Kuo concluded that "a low-fat diet may well be useful in the management of patients with angina."

Arthur Williams, M.D., gave ten angina patients a typical American breakfast of fried eggs, ham, buttered toast and coffee with cream.[20] Four hours later, by examining the small vessels in the patients' eyes, he observed red blood cells sticking together and blocking circulation. He concluded that a high fat meal can lead to the stoppage of blood flow, as observed in eye vessels, and thus cause anginal discomfort by the same mechanism.

Coincidentally, Meyer Friedman, M.D., produced similar results on volunteer firemen, using polyunsaturated oils, in this case, safflower oil.[21] The firemen's red blood cells couldn't tell the difference between animal fats and vegetable oils. The vegetable oils caused clumping and oxygen starvation just as did the saturated fats.

Another way to breach the protective endothelial barrier is by *mechanical* means, such as bashing it with a catheter (accidentally of course) during surgery or during an operative examination.[22] Also the constant twisting and stretching of the coronary arteries in the normal life activity of the heart pumping blood can damage endothelial linings. In either event, the damage will heal normally under conditions of ideal cholesterol levels. However, in the presence of cholesterol levels exceeding 200 mg%, the problem can gradually balloon into a dangerous plaque.[23]

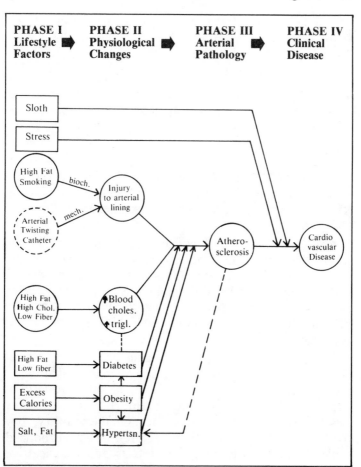

FIG. 8.6:
Diet Lifestyle—Heart Model (Simplified) relating cardiovascular disease to the presence of risk factors.

Some kind of injury to the endothelial layer appears to be a prerequisite for atherosclerotic plaque formation. This endothelial damage is brought about by a shortage of oxygen (or possibly by cholesterol itself) in the blood as a result of smoking and/or a high fat diet, or by mechanical means.

Regardless of the mode of damage, it is usually only in the presence of excess cholesterol in the blood (and aggravated by hypertension) that plaque can form and grow—eventually leading to the heart attack, stroke or other cardiovascular disorder. While elevated blood cholesterol levels are crucial in the plaque building, blood cholesterol levels below 160 mg% are necessary to prevent this process.

Prevention vs. Repair

PREVENTING the disease seems a logical answer. But prevention is often difficult, slow, boring and dull. REPAIR, in contrast, seems quick, exciting and glamorous! Isn't it?

Americans believe in medical repair kits. We build and fill medicine cabinets in our bathroom walls. We have pill boxes in our purses, cars, and attache cases, and on our bedside stands and breakfast tables. Soon, we will need a doctor's medical bag to carry around the burgeoning number of medications that are becoming available for every possible contingency.

Take atherosclerosis, for instance. There are several cholesterol lowering drugs. Big, expensive investigations of these drugs report success in reducing blood cholesterol by levels of five to ten percent.[24-26] Unfortunately, none of these drugs improved life expectancy. On the contrary, they proved more harmful than helpful. They produced unpleasant and distressing side effects and an excessive mortality.[27]

Following the completion of the Coronary Drug Project, evaluating the most popular cholesterol-lowering drugs, the medical journal *Lancet* reported: "The results are depressing for doctors who hoped that a daily pill would improve prognosis, and the results are discouraging for the pharmaceutical industry which has done so much to encourage clinical studies of cholesterol-lowering drugs."[28]

The most glamorous part of the repair kit involves spectacular operations. You have problems? Line up here for your bypass. Or over there for a "rotor-rooter" clean out of your carotid arteries. Or down there for a femoral graft. Quick fixes for life-threatening problems.

In many cases some results have been spectacular. But as time goes on, and statistics accumulate, it's becoming apparent that in the majority of cases these operations do not prolong life, or even necessarily improve it. Short of drastic lifestyle changes, the help is at best temporary.

"The drug costs to save the lives of ten men was $15 million."

Another aspect of the repair kit involves money. One long-term study demonstrated significant benefits of a drug called cholestyramine (Questran).[29] This drug lowered blood cholesterol (when compared to the control group taking a placebo) by 8.5 percent and reduced coronary mortality by 19 percent. This seven-year study involved 3,000 patients and was credited with saving the lives of 10 men. The drug costs alone amounted to $15 million, or about $1.5 million per life saved (!). Surgical approaches are also expensive, averaging around $50,000 per bypass operation. If these trends continue, the repair kit approach may price itself right out of the market.

Today, the glamor and excitement of repair is wearing thin. It has not significantly improved the quantity and quality of life. On the whole, it's been frustrating, disappointing, uncomfortable, inconvenient, temporary and expensive.[30]

There Must be a Better Way

We have a solution. It works as a "repair tool." It can be used to prevent clogged arteries, as well as to help clean them out. And it will cost practically nothing—the price of a healthful home-cooked meal. We suggest *The Monkey Diet,* the diet we named (with tongue-in-cheek) for some simian friends who eat better than we do. (Those great apes are vegetarian, you know.)

Monkeys and Atherosclerosis

The evidence so far is impressive and incriminating, but it's largely circumstantial. It doesn't prove beyond a shadow of a doubt that diet causes heart disease. To do that, researchers needed to find perfectly healthy hearts with clean coronary arteries, and then "create" heart attacks under diet-controlled conditions. The problem: where to find *volunteers* ?

None being forthcoming, research scientists began searching for animals that closely simulate human physiology. They finally selected rhesus monkeys.

Monkeys are hardly "volunteers," but their contribution to heart research is incalculable. To say that many of us owe our lives to research animals like the rhesus monkey is not an overstatement.

In their own habitat, monkeys eat better than we do. Their natural diet consists of fruit, nuts, berries, and grains. And they don't have heart attacks. Forced to give up their monkey diet, however, things begin to change rapidly.

Dr. Taylor and his colleagues became the first team to feed a monkey to death. After being fed typically prepared American food for 2½ years, the rhesus monkey died of a massive heart attack![31] When Dr. Taylor and his colleagues examined the monkey's heart and coronary arteries, they found damage identical to that found in human hearts and coronary arteries after a serious heart attack. They found heart muscle damage and coronary arteries filled with plaque.

"If you want to produce coronary artery disease in monkeys, all you have to do is feed them an average hospital diet."

In his landmark studies with rhesus monkeys, Robert Wissler, M.D., demonstrated again and again that the typical American diet raises blood cholesterol levels and produces significant atherosclerotic plaque. After simulating human plaques in various species for more than twenty years, Dr. Wissler said, "Animal experiments show that no species is immune to atherosclerosis once sustained elevation of (blood) cholesterol has been accomplished."[32]

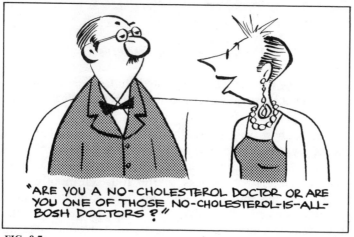

"ARE YOU A NO-CHOLESTEROL DOCTOR OR ARE YOU ONE OF THOSE NO-CHOLESTEROL-IS-ALL-BOSH DOCTORS?"

FIG. 8.7:
The Cholesterol "Controversy"

An eminent cardiologist and researcher at the University of Oregon, William Connor, M.D., stated, "If ever a human disease can be produced in animals, it is atherosclerosis. And if ever the requirements for this disease have been isolated, they are fat and cholesterol in the diet."

Still another researcher, Marc Armstrong, M.D., of the University of Iowa, put a group of thirty rhesus monkeys on a forty percent fat, very high cholesterol diet, increasing their blood cholesterol from 140 mg% to 700 mg%.[33] After seventeen months, ten of the monkeys were sacrificed and their coronary arteries were evaluated. The average artery was sixty percent closed due to atherosclerotic plaque.

He then put some of the remaining animals on a low-fat, cholesterol-free diet. Their blood cholesterol returned to a perfectly normal 140 mg% and in a matter of months the arterial plaque melted away. *It regressed!* It disappeared.

The results of all such experiments in animals are essentially the same. High fat, high cholesterol diets produce high levels of cholesterol in the blood and cause heart disease. Low fat, low cholesterol diets reduce blood cholesterol levels and permit plaque regression.[11, 34-36]Beyond a shadow of a doubt.

Humans and Atherosclerosis

Although the evidence suggested that atherosclerosis is reversible in humans as well, additional research was needed to prove the point.

Drs. Robert Barndt and David Blankenhorn of the University of Southern California used computer techniques to analyze angiographic images of 25 patients with severely blocked arteries in their legs.[37] After fourteen months on a reduced fat and cholesterol-lowering drug program, 9 of the patients showed clear signs of plaque regression, the atherosclerosis had begun to reverse, while plaque build-up continued in the others. What was wrong with the others? Their average cholesterol had dropped only 6 percent, while that of the patients whose atherosclerosis regressed had dropped 21 percent.

"The problem is you've got to be a monkey to get proper treatment for heart disease in this country."
William Castelli, M.D.

Nathan Pritikin, the most outspoken advocate of diet therapy in the management of circulatory disease, proved in his own death that atherosclerosis is indeed reversible.[38] Twenty-five years ago he learned that his own coronary arteries were seriously obstructed. Through a rigorous program of diet and exercise, Pritikin was able to reduce his cholesterol level from over 300 mg% to between 100-130 mg%, and to keep it there for 25 years. The pathologist who performed his autopsy was astounded to find the arteries of a nine-year-old boy in the 69-year-old man. They were "whistle" clean. (See pages 192, 193.)

When Dr. William Castelli (of the Framingham Study) was asked what he thought about the reversibility of atherosclerosis he said, "We have seen many cases of plaque regression in humans. We also know that atherosclerosis can be turned on and off in monkeys with diet. The problem is you've got to be a monkey to get proper treatment for heart disease in this country!"[39]

"The scientific evidence is clear and growing daily stronger: human atherosclerotic plaques, even fibrotic ones, are reversible. Although many clinicians are still skeptical about this, there is little doubt in the minds of researchers."

Cholesterol: Low—Lower—Lowest

If you seriously want to prevent, retard or reverse the insidious progression of atherosclerosis, your blood cholesterol level must come down to 160 mg% or below.[40, 41, 50] Here is the safe and effective way to get it:

Low . . .

Limit the cholesterol in your diet to 100 mg or less per day.

Lower . . .

Reduce your total fat intake to 15 percent of your total daily calories.

Lowest . . .

Eat mostly natural plant foods. Unprocessed foods-as-grown provide energy and endurance, and their natural fiber helps to lower blood cholesterol.

But how about the normal cholesterol needs of the body? The liver and other parts of your body synthesize about 500 mg of cholesterol a day, which is more than enough to meet your needs. A typical American diet, however, provides an additional 500 to 800 mg per day. Much of this excess is processed by the liver, stored for a while in the gall bladder, then passed through the intestines and out in the stool. Unfortunately, the body is limited in its ability to remove large amounts of cholesterol, and the excess accumulates in arteries and other tissues where it can create havoc over the years.

Dietary cholesterol is found exclusively in animal foods. Animals produce their own cholesterol, just as we do. When we eat animals or their products, such as milk, cheese, butter and eggs, we get redundant supplies of cholesterol, much more than our human bodies demand or can safely handle. There is no cholesterol in the plant kingdom, however. Fruits, vegetables, grains and nuts are totally free of cholesterol.

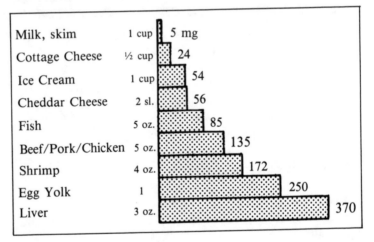

Milk, skim	1 cup	5 mg
Cottage Cheese	½ cup	24
Ice Cream	1 cup	54
Cheddar Cheese	2 sl.	56
Fish	5 oz.	85
Beef/Pork/Chicken	5 oz.	135
Shrimp	4 oz.	172
Egg Yolk	1	250
Liver	3 oz.	370

FIG. 8.8:
Cholesterol Content (in mg) in Selected Foods. Cholesterol is only found in animal products.

What are the sources of cholesterol in the American diet? (See Table 8.2)

Notice that egg yolks account for 35 percent of the cholesterol eaten in America. The percentage is actually higher than that considering baked goods (8% of the total)

Foods	% of total Cholesterol
Meats, poultry, fish	35
Egg yolk	35
Dairy products	16
Commercially baked goods	8
Table & cooking fats	6
	100

TABLE 8.2:
Sources of Dietary Cholesterol (US 1986)

which get most of their cholesterol from eggs used in baking. A three-egg omelette, even without bacon, contains 825 mg of cholesterol (the equivalent to that found in two pounds of hamburger). It's safer to let eggs do what eggs were meant to do: hatch chicks.*

Whole milk and cheese can really push up the cholesterol in your system. ("Vegetarians" who overindulge in eggs and dairy products can actually have higher blood cholesterols than meat eaters!)

Beef, pork, chicken and fish account for another 35 percent of the cholesterol in the American diet. Americans eat an average of 500-800 mg cholesterol per day. If you can lower this to 100 mg per day, your blood cholesterol level will drop *25 points,* and you will reduce your risk of heart attack by *25 percent.*[49]

In addition to reducing the cholesterol in your diet, it is important to lower your total fat intake, and especially the saturated fats which have a powerful effect on blood cholesterol.

*"Lowering your daily intake of cholesterol from 600 to 100 mg will drop your blood cholesterol 25 points. In addition, lowering your daily intake of **saturated fat** from 50 to 15 gm will drop your blood cholesterol 50 points."*

*Only "the incredible edible" **egg white** contains no fat or cholesterol.

Fats: Saturated, Unsaturated and Unsatisfactory

All excess fats are a burden on the body.

• Saturated fats are mostly found in meats and dairy products. They prominently increase the amount of cholesterol in the blood.

• Polyunsaturated fats are said to lower blood cholesterol, but be careful. Polyunsaturated fats are double-edged swords. These fats contribute to overweight, gallstone formation, and recent studies suggest they may be involved in breast and colon cancer.[42-44]

• Excess fat thickens the blood and clumps the blood cells. This reduces oxygen transport, slows circulation and can lead to blocked vessels causing body cells to be starved for oxygen and may be prominently involved in the development of atherosclerosis.[19-21, 45]

• All fats, including vegetable oils, promote the growth of tumors in animals.[46-48]

• High-fat, low-fiber diets contribute to the development of adult onset (Type II) diabetes. (See chapter 6)

• And excess fat in the diet, not surprisingly, is a prime cause of obesity.

Now is the time to cut back or cut out most of the fats in your diet. Remember that most of the dietary fat we eat is hidden—red meat is the single largest source of fat in the American diet (see Table 8.2, page 107). Use oils and hardened fats very sparingly. You really don't need them since a natural food diet easily meets our daily requirements for fat and fatty acids.

By reducing your **saturated** fat intake to 15 grams a day (the American average is 50 grams), you can lower your blood cholesterol *40 to 50 points* and you can reduce your risk of heart disease by almost *50 percent!*[49]

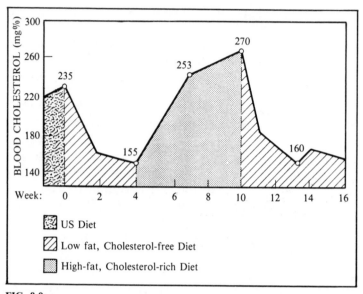

FIG. 8.9:
Diet and Blood Cholesterol Levels
Blood cholesterol can be modified with diet in weeks!

Fabulous Fiber

But everything isn't "doom and gloom" on the food front. You don't have to give up everything, only the bad stuff. There's plenty of good food left to eat, . . . you better believe it! Natural, unrefined, unprocessed food—fruit, vegetables, legumes and whole grain products—these things are good for you, and they all taste great! And natural foods supply one magnificent extra: fiber. It comes on the dinner.

Among other things, you'll be on the move again, naturally, without laxatives or stool "softeners." Fiber also offers considerable protection against appendicitis, hemorrhoids, diverticulosis and, to some extent, varicose veins. Along with its healthier bulk, fiber also traps extra fat, cholesterol and certain other harmful substances that get into our gut. Fiber helps stabilize blood sugar levels, and may protect against colon cancer. Fiber is almost magical stuff.[50]

We Americans today eat about one-fourth the amount of fiber we were eating at the turn of the century when there was less heart disease and colon cancer. The low incidence of these diseases among the Japanese and other peoples of the earth may be a reflection of their relatively high fiber diet.

IN SUMMARY: Blood cholesterol is directly affected by the richness of your diet. If you don't know what your blood cholesterol level is, run, don't walk, to the nearest checkpoint. The procedure takes less than five minutes in your doctor's office or in the laboratory. Use the results as a motivator and a guide to improve your dietary lifestyle. If your cholesterol level is over 160 mg%, it's time to get serious about "The Monkey Diet."

That natural solution for lowering Blood Cholesterol and Triglycerides* involves

1. SEVERELY LIMIT CHOLESTEROL—avoid all animal products, such as meat, sausages, egg yolks, liver, dairy products (unless they are low or non-fat products). If you use fish and fowl, use them sparingly.

2. SUBSTANTIALLY REDUCE ALL SATURATED FATS—avoid saturated fats, which are mainly found in animal products (covered under guideline #1) and in palm and coconut oil.

3. GET DOWN TO YOUR IDEAL WEIGHT—avoid highly refined, empty calorie foods, low in fiber. (See page 52.) This includes the visible fats and oils, sugar and alcohol. Use nuts only sparingly.

4. EAT PLENTY OF UNREFINED STARCHY FOODS, FRESH FRUITS AND VEGETABLES—eat all you want of the unrefined whole grain products, of legumes and of fresh vegetables and fruits. And enjoy those potatoes, yams and sweet potatoes! These foods not only satisfy, but are also rich in fiber.

---

*The major cause of high triglycerides in 80 percent of cases is obesity. Get down to your ideal weight by avoiding fats and sugars. (Triglyceride-sensitive persons may need to limit even natural sugar-containing products, such as fruit juices, apple sauces, canned fruits, and dehydrated fruits like raisins and dates.) Also avoid alcohol and control diabetes (see page 66).

5. WALK DAILY—a regular exercise program can further help in lowering your blood cholesterol somewhat. At the same time, it may improve your HDL portion of your cholesterol, which appears protective.

6. SEE YOUR PHYSICIAN—your physician is in a position to rule out any *unusual* causes of high cholesterol levels. Your physician can prescribe cholesterol lowering drugs, if the lifestyle approach needs to be complemented. But remember: the *safest* way to reduce your blood cholesterol is through dietary means. Drugs are a last resort. And try to get your blood pressure under control, hopefully without the cholesterol-elevating diuretic drugs (see page 78).

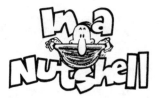

℞ How to Lower Your Blood Cholesterol

1. *Severely Limit Cholesterol*—avoid all animal products, such as meats, eggs and dairy (unless low or non-fat products)

2. *Severely Reduce Saturated Fats*—reduce saturated fat by especially avoiding animal products

3. *Get Down to Your Ideal Weight*

4. *Eat Plenty of Natural Plant Foods*

5. *Walk Daily*

6. *See Your Physician*—if possible, replace diuretic drugs. If necessary, use cholesterol-lowering medication.

Bibliography—Chapter 8

[1] Kannel, W.B. et al. (1971) The Framingham Study. *Ann Intern Med* 74:1-12. See also
Rosenman, R.H. et al. (1967) Comparative predicted value of three serum lipid entries in a prospective study of ischemic heart disease. *Circulation* 35, Suppl. 2.

[2] McGill, H.C. (1968) The geographic pathology of atherosclerosis. *Lab Invest* 18:463-478.

[3] Welch, C.C. et al. (1970) Cinecoronary arteriography in young men. *Circulation* 62:625-631.

[4] Page, I.H. et al. (1970) Prediction of coronary heart disease based on chemical suspicion, age, total cholesterol and triglycerides. *Circulation* 42:625-645.

[5] Keys, A. (1970) Coronary heart disease in seven countries. *Circulation* 41, Suppl. 1.

[6] Keys, A. et al. (1958) Lessons from serum cholesterol studies in Japan, Hawaii, and Los Angeles. *Ann Intern Med* 48:83-94. (See also 1976—61:421-430.)

[7] Stamler, J. (1978) Lifestyles, major risk factors, proof and public policy. *Circulation* 58:3-19.

[8] Gotto, A. (1977) *Hearings before the Select Committee on Nutrition and Human Needs of the US Senate.* Part I, CVD—Diet related to killer diseases, II. pp. 325-326.

[9] Gotto, A. (1977) quoted in *New West*, Feb. 4.

[10] Castelli, W. (1979) quoted in *Med World News*, Sept. 3.

[11] Barnard, R.J. et al. (1983) Effects of an intensive exercise and nutrition program on patients with coronary artery disease: a 5-year follow-up. *J Card Rehab* 3(3):183-190.

[12] Castelli, W. P. et al. (1986) Incidence of Coronary Heart Disease and Lipoprotein Cholesterol Levels. The Framingham Study. *JAMA:* 256:235-238.

[13] Wright, I.S. (1976) Editorial: Correct levels of serum cholesterol: average vs. normal vs. optimal. *JAMA.* 236:261-262.

[14] Ross, R. and J. A. Glomset. (1976) The pathogenesis of atherosclerosis, parts 1 and 2. *N Engl J Med* 295:369-375 and 420-426.

[15] Ross, R. (1982) Lipoproteins, endothelial injury and atherosclerosis. *Cardiovasc Res Rep* 3:1026-1033.

[16] Astrup, P. (1973) Carbon monoxide, smoking and cardiovascular disease. *Circulation* 48:1167-1168.

[17] Wells, R. E. (1964) Rheology of blood in the microvasculature. *N Engl J Med* 270:832-839.

[18] Swank, R.D. and H. Nakamura. (1960) Oxygen availability in brain tissues after lipid meals. *Am J Physiol.* 198:217-220.

[19] Kuo, P.T. and C.R. Joyner. (1955) Angina pectoris induced by fat ingestion in patients with coronary artery disease. *JAMA* 158:1008-1012.

[20] Williams, A.V. et al. (1957) Increased cell agglutination following ingestion of fat, a factor contributing to cardiac ischemia, coronary insufficiency and anginal pain. *Angiology* 8:29-36.

[21] Friedman, M. et al. (1965) Effect of unsaturated fats upon lipemia and conjunctival circulation. *JAMA* 193:882-886.

[22] Ross, R. and L. Harker. (1976) Hyperlipidemia and atherosclerosis. *Science* 193:1094-1100.

[23] Glagov, S. (1972) Hemodynamic risk factors. (Eds.) Wissler, R.W. and J.C. Greer in: *The pathogenesis of atherosclerosis.* Baltimore, Williams & Wilkins. pp. 164-199.

[24] Ahrens, E.H. (1976) The management of hyperlipidemia: whether, rather than how. *Ann Intern Med* 85:87-93.

[25] Editorial (1978) *Brit Med J* 2:1585-1586.

[26] Rifkind, B.M. and R.I. Levy. (1978) Testing the Lipid hypothesis. *Arch Surg* 113:80-83.

[27] Coronary Drug Project Research Group (1975) Clofibrate and niacin in coronary heart disease. *JAMA* 231:360-381.

[28] Lipid-lowering Drugs after M.I. (1975) Editorial *Lancet I:* 501-502.

[29] The Lipid Research Clinics Coronary Primary Prevention Trial Results (1984) *JAMA* 251:351-374.

[30] Diehl, H.A. and D. Mannerberg. (1981) Regression of certain Western diseases. (Eds.) H. Trowell and D. Burkitt. *Western Diseases: their emergence and prevention.* London. Edward Arnold (Publ.) Ltd. pp. 392-411.

[31] Taylor, C.B. et al. (1963) Atherosclerosis in rhesus monkeys. *Arch Path* 76:404-409.

[32] Wissler, R.W. et al. (1965) Aortic lesions and blood lipids in rhesus monkeys fed "table prepared" human diets. *Circulation,* Suppl. 2.

[33] Armstrong, M.L. et al. (1970) Regressing coronary atheromatosis in rhesus monkeys. *Circ Res* 27:59-67.

114 / To Your Health

[34] Tucker, C. et al. (1971) Regression of cholesterol-induced atherosclerotic lesions in rhesus monkeys. *Circulation* 63, Suppl. 2.

[35] Vesselinovitch, D. et al. (1976) Reversal of advanced atherosclerosis in rhesus monkeys. *Atheroscl.* 23:155-176.

[36] Bond, M.G. (1976) The effect of plasma cholesterol concentrations on regression of primate atherosclerosis. *Am J Path* (abst.) 82:69a.

[37] Barndt, R. and D.H. Blankenhorn. (1977) Regression and progression of early femoral atherosclerosis in treated hyperlipoproteinemic patients. *Ann Intern Med* 86:139-143.

[38] Hubbard, J.D. et al. (1985) Nathan Pritikin's heart. *N Engl J Med* 313:52-53.

[39] Monte, T. (1980) quoting W. Castelli in *Nutrition Action,* April pp. 3-7.

[40] Pritikin, N. (1982) Optimal Dietary Recommendations: A Public Health Responsibility. *Prev Med* 11:733-739.

[41] Stamler, J. et al. (1986) Is Relationship Between Serum Cholesterol and Risk of Premature Death From Coronary Heart Disease Continuous and Graded? The MRFIT Study. *JAMA* 256:2823-2828.

[42] Nestel, P. (1973) Lowerings of plasma cholesterol and enhanced sterol excretion with the consumption of polyunsaturated ruminant fats. *N Engl J Med* 299:1221-1225.

[43] Bennion, L. (1978) Risk factors for the development of cholelithiasis in man. *N Engl J Med* 299:1221-1225.

[44] Broitman, S. (1977) Polyunsaturated fat, cholesterol and tumorigenesis. *Cancer* 40:2455-2459.

[45] Cullen, C. (1954) Intravascular aggregation and adhesiveness of the blood elements associated with alimentary lipemia and injections of large molecular substances. *Circulation* 9:335-339.

[46] Carroll, K. (1975) Experimental evidence of dietary factors and hormone-dependent cancers. *Cancer Res* 35:3374-3379.

[47] Hill, P. (1977) Diet and endocrine-related cancer. *Cancer* 39:1820-1824.

[48] Nishizuka, Y. (1978) Biological influence of fat intake on mammary cancer and mammary tissue: experimental correlates. *Prev Med* 7:218-223.

[49] Grundy, S.M. (1986) Cholesterol and Coronary Heart Disease: A New Era. *JAMA* 256:2849-2858.

[50] Hammond, H.K. (1983) Regression of Atherosclerosis—A Review. *J Cardiac Rehab* 3:347-359.

[51] Majno, G. et al. (1984) The diet/atherosclerosis connection: new insights. *J Cardiovasc. Med.* Jan. 21-28.

Diet and Disease:
Summary and Recommendations

Desirable and Dangerous

The American diet, rich in meat, eggs, dairy products, sweets, ice cream, pastries and fried foods, is the envy of much of the world. This kind of diet has been regarded as a desirable diet on which our children can grow strong and big. However, our present American diet is at great variance with human dietary traditions. The Babylonians and the Hebrews, the Egyptians, Greeks and Romans built their cultures on diets of wheat. The Oriental cultures built theirs on diets of rice. The Aztecs and Mayas built their cultures on the dietary staples of corn and beans. These great civilizations developed with the people consuming largely whole grain foods, fruits, vegetables and legumes.

Meat in those cultures was reserved for *special feast days,* or it was used as seasoning. At the same time, sugar, fat and salt in the absence of chemical and food technology was very scarce. Even in Western culture only the affluent, until recently, had the means to eat a meat-and-animal-product-centered diet. Bread and potatoes were the basic foods most people used.

However, with economic prosperity and food technology it is now possible for most of us to feast *every day.*

Inexpensive starchy foods such as whole wheat bread, potatoes and grains no longer serve as the "staff of life" for the masses. Rather, most grain is now set aside as fodder to fatten animals for the human larder. Thus animal products, such as meat and poultry, eggs and dairy products, and fats consumed as spreads, cooking oils and salad dressings have become staples of the masses. Most of the people, not just the elite, live off the fat of the land. By historic standards, the dietary shift is staggering.

"Rich diet is the major cause of death and disability in the United States."

It is this rich diet, which affluent people generally consume, that is everywhere associated with similar disease patterns: high rates of heart disease, stroke, hypertension, diabetes, certain forms of cancer and obesity. These are the major causes of death and disability in the United States. In no race for which a high cholesterol and high fat intake is recorded, is atherosclerosis, cardiovascular disease and most cancers absent.

An interesting confirmation of this international observation is provided by an American population group, the Seventh-day Adventists. Members of this conservative religious group do not smoke and consume less animal fat and cholesterol. Their age-adjusted death rates for cancer and cardiovascular disease are considerably lower than those of the general population. However, most interestingly, a carefully standardized 20-year follow-up study among Adventists in California found significantly different rates for fatal heart disease among Adventist groups, which differentiated themselves most and uniquely in their consumption of animal products (see Figure 9.1). The lowest death rate was found among Adventist total vegetarians, then among lacto-ovo vegetarians (dairy and egg consuming "vegetarians"), and then the meat-eating Adventists. The highest rate was found in matched controls of Californians, who often were also smokers.

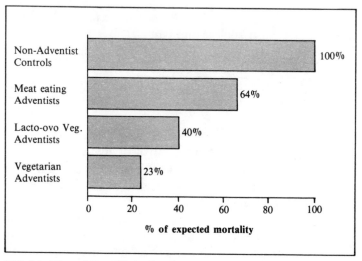

FIG. 9.1: Diet and Fatal Heart Attack

Japanese who migrate to the United States and change to a Western diet from their traditional Japanese diet (which contains only 10-15% fat, and almost no dairy and meat products) dramatically increase their incidence of cardiovascular disease, breast and colon cancer, clearly deemphasizing the etiological role of racial genetics.

It is therefore reasonable to incriminate the "rich" diet as the *primary, essential and necessary cause* of the current epidemic of atherosclerotic diseases and a majority of cancers.

Diet Change and Disease

A massive body of scientific evidence shows that these modern, Western killer diseases are largely the result of our lifestyle, especially the way we eat. As such, these diseases are substantially preventable and reversable. The question to be asked is not "why *should* we change?" but "why *shouldn't* we change towards a simpler, more plant-food centered diet?" What are the risks associated with eating *less* meat and cholesterol, less fat, sugar and salt and instead eating *more* fresh fruits and vegetables, potatoes, beans and whole grain products? There is none that can be identified. On the contrary: such a diet can

1. substantially reduce blood cholesterol and triglyceride levels in as little as four weeks.
2. reduce or totally eliminate the need for insulin injections in adult onset diabetics without spilling sugar in the urine.
3. replace many of the drugs (and their side effects) presently used for the control of hypertension.
4. markedly reduce the risk of colon cancer and large bowel disease, probably because of its high fiber and low fat content.
5. ease the problem of weight control and constipation. The high fiber content of fresh fruits and vegetables and the bulk of whole grains and beans can bring satiety and satisfaction of appetite more readily than do highly refined foods.
6. become good medicine for ailing food budgets.

Dietary Goals for the United States

After a detailed study and years of testimony from the leading scientists in the world, the United States Select Committee on Nutrition and Human Needs published *Dietary Goals for the United States* advising Americans to double their intake of starchy foods, and to cut their consumption of sugar, total fat (especially saturated fats), cholesterol and salt by 30 to 50 percent.[1]

These government issued guidelines have been reinforced by recent dietary guidelines from the National Cancer Institute for the prevention of cancer. Ernst Wynder, M.D., president of the American Health Foundation and a highly respected scientist, has estimated that 50 percent of all the major cancers in the Western world, such as those of the colon, prostate, uterus and breast, relate to over-nutrition, especially to the excesses of fat and cholesterol.

This concern about diet and cancer was amplified by the Surgeon General's Report on Health Promotion and Disease Prevention (1979). The Surgeon General stated that the high consumption of animal protein and the excessive intake of fat, both from animal **and** vegetable sources, may be directly linked to colon and breast cancer.[2]

"Fifty percent of all major cancers relate to excesses of fat, cholesterol, and calories, another 30 percent to smoking. Dietary excess and smoking relate to 80 percent of America's major cancers. What we need is not better treatment, but a health-enhancing lifestyle."

Optimal Diet

The importance of the U.S. Dietary Goals does not reside so much in its content as in the fact that it was the first major bipartisan effort delineating the dietary relationship to chronic killer diseases and to making it publicly known. Although the advocated changes were moderate, they elicited strong reactions. Consumer advocates hailed the Dietary Goals as a major breakthrough towards improving health, while the food lobbies and the American Medical Association condemned them as being prematurely conceived. It was very clear: this historic report aimed at improving national health would usher in a turning away from the rich American diet and a turning towards a somewhat simpler diet. Major political and economic changes and alignments were in the making . . .

The Dietary Goals were reasonable and sound as a **first** step towards health improvement. For instance, they recommended a lowering of total fat from 42 percent of calories to 30 percent. (See Table 9.1.) At the same time the authors suggested that further reductions may be desirable:

"There is increasing research that suggests that some day a dietary fat intake of 20 percent to 25 percent might be recommended, and even less for those people who already have heart disease. The basic research is strongly corroborated by studies of populations throughout the world who live quite well on a diet containing as little as 10 percent calories from fat."[1]

Dr. Diehl's Dietary Decalogue

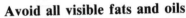

Avoid all visible fats and oils

Avoid fatty meals, cooking and salad oils, dressings and shortening. Use margarine and nuts only very sparingly. Avoid frying wherever and whenever possible—instead saute with water or use fine film of lecithin.

Avoid all sugars

Avoid sugar, honey, molasses, syrups, pies, cakes, pastries, candy, cookies, soft drinks and sugar-rich desserts (jello, pudding, ice cream, etc.)

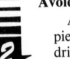

Severely limit cholesterol

Avoid all cholesterol containing foods such as: meat, sausages, egg yolks, liver, dairy products (except low fat or non fat products—ex. replace whole milk with skim; replace creamed cottage cheese with low fat cottage cheese; replace cheddar cheese with Farmer's or Hoop cheese). If you use fish and fowl, use them sparingly.

Severely limit salt

Don't salt your plate or cooking pot. Avoid obviously salty products like dill pickles, crackers, soy sauce, salted popcorn, nuts, pretzels, chips and garlic salt.

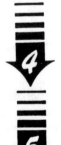

Avoid alcohol, black tea, caffeinated drinks

Dr. Diehl's Dietary Decalogue

6

Freely use whole grain products

Freely use brown rice, millet, barley, whole wheat bread, oatmeal, corn, cracked wheat, whole wheat spaghetti, shredded wheat, etc.

7

Freely use tubers and legumes

Freely use potatoes (but without the liberal "toppings"), sweet potatoes, yams, squash, lentils, beans, peas, etc.

8

Freely use fruits and vegetables

Freely eat fresh fruits in season. Avoid canned fruits in heavy syrups. Limit the use of fruit juices. Freely eat fresh vegetables and salads.

9

Drink plenty of water

Drink at least 8 glasses of (filtered) water or herb teas daily.

10

Eat a good breakfast daily

Don't skip your breakfast, especially if you try to lose weight. A hot multi-grain cereal stabilizes your blood sugar, emotions, and nervous system.

Indeed, half-hearted changes in diet are not enough to turn the epidemic around. If we want to win the battle against the epidemic of Western lifestyle diseases, then we must break with the American Diet, which is lethal in its excesses. We must adopt a simpler more natural dietary lifestyle, a lifestyle that allows us to eat more, cut our food bill in half and have better and more bouyant health.

"If we want to win the battle against the epidemic of Western lifestyle diseases, then we must break with the American diet, which is lethal in its excesses."

Such a diet should not only prevent Western lifestyle diseases, but be a therapeutic one as well.

Research with therapeutic nutrition has clearly demonstrated a *unitary* dietary principle in dealing with Western killer diseases: there is not a special diet for the treatment of heart disease, another diet for overweight, another for diabetes and yet another for hypertension and high cholesterol levels. Instead, there is *one OPTIMAL DIET*. Such a diet consists of: "A wide variety of foods, freely eaten 'as grown,' simply prepared with sparing use of fats and oils, sugars, and salt, and almost devoid of refined processed foods. If animal products are eaten, they should be used as seasoning."

Such a more natural diet will be very low in fat (ideally under 15 percent) and very low in cholesterol (ideally under 100 mg/day). At the same time, such a diet encourages liberal intake of unrefined complex carbohydrates, which are high in fiber and bulk, thus making weight gain rather difficult. (See Table 9.1.)

It is this kind of a diet that will not only prevent Western diseases, but it has been demonstrated to be effective as **the** major therapeutic factor in regressing disease and *restoring* a higher level of health. If you follow these dietary guidelines, you can add more life to your years and healthy years to your life.

| | U.S. DIET | COMPARISON | |
		U.S. DIETARY GOALS	OPTIMAL DIET
Fats and Oils	42%*	30%	15%
Complex Carbohyd.	22%	42%	60-65%
Refined Sugar	18%	10%	minimal
Cholesterol/day	500 mg	300 mg	100 mg
Salt/day	15-20 gm	5 gm	5 gm
Fiber/day	10-15 gm		40-60 gm
Water (Fluids)			8 glasses/day
*of total calories			

TABLE 9.1 Dietary Comparison: US Diet, US Dietary Goals, Optimal Diet

TO YOUR HEALTH!

We have given you a lot to chew on—much more than you asked for, perhaps—and certainly more than we hinted in our television series. We hope this will be the beginning of your new lifestyle.

In the following pages you'll find directions, recipes and guides to help you change your dietary lifestyle. Only you can make a committed choice in favor of better health. But don't let it be a lonely journey. Take your family with you, slowly at first to be sure, but as they gradually taste and experience the better life, they'll not only one day appreciate your leading the way, they will help you eat and drink "To Your Health!"

---

[1] Dietary Goals for the U.S. (1977) Washington, D.C., US Gov. Printing Office, No. 052-070-04376-8.

[2] Surgeon General (1979) *Report on Health Promotion and Disease Prevention.* Washington, D.C., US Gov. Printing Office.

Dietary Guidelines

THE OPTIMAL DIET

FOODS TO USE and *FOODS TO AVOID*

FATS:
  Keep to an absolute minimum.
  Avoid butter, margarine, shortening, lard, meat fat, all oils.

EGGS:
  Egg white only.
  Avoid egg yolk, fish eggs (caviar)

DAIRY PRODUCTS:
  Nonfat or skim milk, evaporated skim milk, buttermilk, nonfat yogurt, 100% skim milk cheese, hoop cheese, dry curd cottage cheese, lowfat cottage cheese.

  Avoid whole milk, lowfat milk, sour cream, cream, half-and-half, non-dairy creamers, whipped cream, ice cream, pasteurized cheeses, cream cheese.

FLESH FOODS (if you insist):
Poultry without the skin, fish fillets, lean beef (no more than 3 ounces three times per week)
Avoid pork, lamb, organ meats, luncheon meats, sausages, bacon, frozen and packaged dinners, shellfish. Preferably, do not use poultry, fish and beef. If you do, use it as seasoning.

BEANS AND PEAS:
Use freely all beans, peas, lentils, garbanzos.
Avoid soybean-based meat substitutes or use them sparingly.

TUBERS:
Use freely potatoes, yams, sweet potatoes, roots.
Avoid fatty toppings.

VEGETABLES:
Use freely.
Avoid those prepared with butter, cheese, cream sauces. Use avocado and olives sparingly only.

GRAINS:
Use freely all *whole* grains: breads, cereals, crackers, pasta, tortillas that are low in fat and salt. Try oats, millet, barely rye, cracked wheat, 7-grain cereal, brown rice, etc.
Limit refined grain products, such as white flour, white rice, whole pasta, white bread. Avoid gluten-based meat substitutes, or use them sparingly.

NUTS AND SEEDS:
Use sparingly.

FRUITS:
Freely use *fresh* fruits. If canned or frozen, use only unsweetened fruits.
Avoid fruits canned in syrup, fruit drinks and punches,

even unsweetened fruit drinks and juices, dried fruits and apple sauces—use them in great moderation.

SUGAR:
Keep to absolute minimum. The less the better.
Avoid as much as possible all extracted sugars, including syrups, honey, molasses, fructose, dextrose, sucrose, etc.

MISCELLANEOUS:
Drink plenty of water, herb teas, mineral water. Use lemon juice, herbs and most spices.
Avoid alcohol and caffeine beverages, sodas, strong spices and keep salt to a minimum.

FOOD SELECTION

As you are planning your new, more natural dietary program, you will want to select from a large variety of foods from this list and eat liberally.

FRUIT: All fresh fruit (avocado & olives sparingly)
VEGETABLES: All vegetables, greens and herbs, squash
LEGUMES: All beans, peas, lentils, garbanzos
TUBERS: Potatoes, yams, sweet potatoes, roots
GRAINS: All **whole** grains, breads, pasta
NUTS: Eat sparingly only
DAIRY:* *Use in moderation:* milk, nonfat cheese, nonfat milk, cheese, plain yogurt, buttermilk, lowfat cottage cheese.
Optional item—EGGS: Egg whites only. Avoid food containing yolks.
If you insist—FLESH FOODS *in small amounts* (3 ounces, 3 times a week): Skinless fowl, fish fillet, lean beef.

To obtain good nutrition in terms of vitamins and minerals (see Appendix, page 194) you will want to eat daily **at least:**

FRUITS: One citrus plus another fresh fruit
VEGETABLES: One serving of green vegetables, one serving of yellow vegetables, one mixed salad
LEGUMES: One serving of beans, peas or lentils
GRAINS: Three servings of different whole grain products
TUBERS: Use as desired
DAIRY*: Skim milk products (1-2 servings)
   * Can be optional for pure vegetarians, but requires more special dietary planning.

SAMPLE MENU FOR A DAY

Here is a sample menu to give you an idea what it could look like. Invent your own sequence of dishes that are most appropriate for you and your family's taste.

Breakfast
- Cooked cereal (7-grain cereal, rolled oats, millet, brown rice, rolled rye, wheat flakes, cracked wheat) or cold cereal (Shredded Wheat, Nutri-grain) with skimmed milk and sliced banada (½) or other fresh fruit.
- Citrus fruit: Orange, grapefruit.
- 2 slices of whole wheat toast with "mashed" banana (½) topped with pineapple ring or slice of Kiwi-fruit.
- Herbal tea.

Lunch
- 2 whole wheat pita (pocket) breads stuffed with lettuce, sprouts, cucumbers, tomatoes, radishes and some lowfat cottage cheese.
- Split pea soup with pearl barley or rice.
- Fresh fruit, such as papaya, pear, apple.

Dinner
- Whole wheat spaghetti noodles with sauce.
- Tossed salad with low-calorie Italian dressing.
- Slice of bread with garbanzo spread.
- For dessert: baked apple (microwaved)

If snack is needed: use fresh fruit, crisp raw vegetables, flat breads.

MOVING *TOWARDS* THE OPTIMAL DIET

Here are some guidelines for streamlining your recipes:

1. Consider whether the amount of oil, margarine, or butter in the recipes can be reduced or even eliminated. For example:

    a. Cook onions and green peppers in a little broth instead of browning in fat; add garlic and herbs to enhance the flavor.

    b. In quick breads, such as muffins, cornbread, and fruit loaves, the fat can frequently be cut in half without affecting the quality of the final product.

    c. Meat can be browned in a non-stick pan (teflon) without adding oil. Cook meat in its own juices and then pour off the drippings. If you use meat, always use very lean and in small amounts—more like a "condiment."

    d. Eliminate the dabs of butter from casserole toppings.

    e. Instead of greasing a casserole dish, use a non-stick spray such as Pam, or a *film* of lecithin (if layer is not thin enough, it may turn brown-black!)

2. In recipes which call for milk, cut calories and cost by using reconstituted nonfat dry milk. In recipes using evaporated milk or light cream, substitute evaporated skim milk.

3. To replace sour cream, use nonfat plain yogurt or blend it with an equal amount of lowfat cottage cheese.

4. If you make stews, chili, and roasts, refrigerate before

serving so the fat will harden and can be removed. Chill meat drippings and remove the fat; then serve your roast *au jus* instead of with gravy. Or make a gravy with fat-free broth, skimmed milk, and flour or cornstarch.

5. Replace an egg with two egg whites.

6. Serve foods more simply. Serve fresh fruits. Serve vegetables *au natural* instead of heavily sauced. These ideas will save you time and money as well as calories.

7. In quick bread, muffin and cookie recipes, the sugar can be cut in half and natural sweeteners such as bananas, dates, raisins, shredded carrots or chopped apple may be used. Extracts such as vanilla, almond or cherry also enhance sweetness.

8. If your recipe calls for cheese, use "hoop" cheese or lowfat cheese and skim milk instead of whole milk.

9. Use herbs, garlic and onions and low calorie dressings to season vegetables instead of butter, bacon, salt and oily dressings.

10. Introduce more oriental dishes.

The worse off you are with cardiovascular disease, diabetes, obesity, etc., the nearer you must aim for the center of the target of a calorie controlled, very low fat, very low cholesterol, high fiber diet.

SUMMARY: Eat a wide variety of "foods as grown," simply prepared with sparing use of fats and oils, sugars and salt. Use refined products and animal products, if used at all, only sparingly.

2

Recipes

GRAINS

Grains are the most abundant foodstuffs in the world. They represent a great array of variety: barley, rye, wheat, oats, corn, buckwheat, millet, brown rice! And there are now 3-, 5-, 7-, 9-grain cereal mixtures available.

Enjoy the abundance of grains. Choose the unrefined form with the intended nutrition intact; don't settle for the refined and "enriched" kind. Grains are an exceptional source of the B-vitamins niacin, riboflavin, thiamin. They are also an excellent source of iron and fiber, and they carry moderate amounts of protein and calcium. They are low in fat and price. Make them one of the main foods in your new diet.

Start the day with a good hot cereal. With some planning, it hardly takes any time. Learn to use your crockpot to benefit you: put your grain of choice with adequate water in your pot, set it on low heat at night before going to bed,

* Recipes used or adapted with permission from publishers are numbered 1-7. The sources are listed on page 202.

and the next morning your breakfast cereal is ready only awaiting your flavoring touches. Or use cold cereals, like Shredded Wheat, Nutri-grains, etc.

Or use the different grains like pearl barley and brown rice to provide extra bulk and nutrition to your vegetable soups. Whole wheat spaghetti, fettucini, pasta and lasagna are delicious dishes. And what about tabouli and whole grain waffles? Or home-baked breads?

Cooking Guide for Grains			
Cups of dry Whole Kernel grain	Water (cups)	Cooking Time	Yield (cups)
1 buckwheat	4	20 mins.	5
1 millet	4	1 hr.	4
1 brown rice	2½	1 hr.	4
1 cracked wheat	4	20 mins.	3
1 barley*	4	1 hr.	4
1 triticale**	3	30 mins.	3½
1 rye*	5	6 hrs.	4½
1 wheat berries*	4	6 hrs.	3
1 whole oats*	3	1 hr.	3

All grains: boil three minutes, then reduce heat to simmer; cover and do not remove lid during cooking time.

When using double-boiler, rice cooker or crockpot, double the cooking time.

For delicious flavor, use the slow thorough cooking methods. Time brings out the flavor in softening the cellulose.

*These grains need to be soaked overnight in cold water.

**Triticale is a cross between wheat and rye.

French Toast (12 slices)

1¼ c. rolled oats
½ c. cashew nuts
1¼ c. orange juice

1 banana
6 dates
1¾ c. water

Blenderize all ingredients until satiny smooth. Pour batter into flat-bottomed bowl. Dip whole wheat bread into batter and brown on both sides in Pam-sprayed skillet over medium-low heat.

Serve with Waffle Topping (see page 133).

Buckwheat-Oat Waffles[3] (5 servings)

2¼ c. water   ½ c. buckwheat flour
1½ c. rolled oats   ¼ c. soy flour
1 Tbsp. oil

Whiz all ingredients in blender until foamy and smooth. Let stand 10 minutes for batter to thicken. Whiz again before pouring batter onto hot Pam-sprayed waffle iron. Bake 10 minutes. (Warning: don't lift lid too soon!)

Serve with waffle toppings (see page 133).

Cashew-Oat Waffles[3] (5 servings)

2¼ c. water   ⅓ c. raw cashew nuts
1½ c. rolled oats   1 Tbsp. oil

Follow the instructions of Buckwheat Waffles.

Multi-Grain Waffles[3]

½ c. rolled oats   ½ c. soy flour
½ c. rye flour   2¼ c. water
½ c. whole wheat flour   1 Tbsp. oil

Follow method in Buckwheat-Oat Waffle recipe.

Whole Berry Crock Cereal (5 cups)

1 c. barley, wheat, or rye berries
½ c. millet or brown rice
5 c. hot tap water

Combine all in crockpot. Bring to boil, then put on low or medium heat and let simmer overnight.

Variation: 20 minutes before serving, stir in ¾ c. dried fruit (chopped), such as apricots, raisins, apple. Or serve with banana milk, blenderizing 3 cups of skim-milk with 5 frozen bananas and 1 tsp. vanilla.

Topping for Pancakes, Toast, and Waffles

1. Mashed bananas with a squeeze of lemon.

2. Raspberries or strawberries.

3. Crushed pineapple or fresh blueberries thickened with some cornstarch.

4. Any canned fruit, such as peaches, apricots, cherries, sweetened with some frozen concentrated apple juice and thickened with cornstarch will make a delicious topping.

Try this: **Pineapple-Orange Topping (makes 6 cups)**

½ c. orange juice concentrate	1½ c. pineapple juice
3 c. unsweetened pineapple chunks	1 small banana
	1 c. water

Whiz together in blender. Heat and thicken with arrowroot, tapioca flour or cornstarch.

Wheat-Oat Crepes (16—6″ crepes)

¾ c. whole wheat pastry flour	¾ c. quick rolled oats
2 c. skim milk	1 tbsp. oil

Whiz all ingredients in blender. Let stand 5 minutes. Heat a small non-stick skillet or crepe pan; apply *thin* layer of lecithin.*

Spoon in 3 tbsp. batter, spread evenly by tilting skillet. Brown lightly on both sides.

Crepes are versatile for any meal, with fillings ranging from Chinese vegetables to fruits.

Fill with: 1. Topping for waffles—toast—pancakes

2. Uncreamed cottage cheese topped off with thickened blueberries or strawberries

3. Chinese bean sprouts

4. Fresh-apple crepe filling: Mix 2 Tbsp. honey with 2 Tbsp. almond butter, lemon juice (1 tsp.) and 2 drops of anise. Add 1½ cups of shredded apple, mix well.

5. Experiment!

*Use mixture of ½ vegetable oil and ½ liquid lecithin. Using just *a few* drops, spread over the entire baking surface of the pan or casserole with fingertips. Then wipe off entire surface *very thoroughly* with a paper towel. Any left on will turn black during cooking. Even though it looks as if there is no lecithin coating left, it provides an excellent release and an easy-to-clean surface. Use for all baking pans and frying pans in place of oil. It works as well as Teflon or Silverstone if pan is not overheated.

Shirley's Millet Loaf (serves 5)

1 c. whole raw millet	5 c. tomato juice (low salt)
1 med. onion	1 can chopped olives
½ tsp. Savory	¼ tsp. sage
4 Tbsp. ground sunflower seeds	

Whiz onion in blender using part of tomato juice. Mix everything in. Pour into a baking dish treated with thin lecithin layer.

Bake in covered casserole or baking pan at 325° for 2 to 3 hours or until liquid is absorbed. Uncover for last 30 mins. to brown lightly, if desired. Garnish with parsley and pineapple rings. If tomato flavor is too strong, substitute one cup of water for one cup of tomato juice.

Millet Vegetable Casserole[2] (9 servings)

1 Tbsp. oil	1 large onion, chopped
1 c. whole raw millet	1 large carrot, sliced
1 c. sliced mushrooms	2 c. water
2 c. McKay's chicken-style broth	1 c. plain nonfat yogurt

Brown millet in oil. Add onions, carrots, mushrooms, water and chicken broth.

Bake at 350° in 2-quart casserole for 1 hour or until most of the liquid is absorbed. Stir once or twice to blend the vegetables and grain. Top with yogurt, garnish with parsley and serve.

Tabouli, a Middle Eastern favorite [6] (serves 6)

This nutritious dish is ideal for hot days, in that it is served chilled. Can be made ahead of time. Keeps well. Terrific!

1 c. uncooked bulgur wheat	2 c. boiling water
2 tomatoes, finely diced	½ c. lemon juice
1 c. parsley, finely chopped	½ c. green onions, chopped
3 Tbsp. fresh mint, chopped	1 c. cooked garbanzos
or 2 tsp. dried mint	¼ tsp. garlic powder

Some 3 hrs. before meal time, place uncooked bulgur wheat in bowl and pour boiling water over bulgur. Cover with towel and let soak for 1 hr. Drain well. Stir in other ingredients and chill for 1-2 hours. Serve garnished with halved cherry tomatoes and lemon slices. Can be used as a grain dish or as a salad, and makes an ideal pita bread stuffing. Leftovers can be added to soup (just add to crockpot ½ hr. before serving)

Spaghetti[7] (serves 8)

1 lb. whole wheat spaghetti

Sauce:

8 c. blended unpeeled and
  fresh tomatoes
4 c. mushrooms, sliced
4 garlic cloves, minced (4 tsp.)
3 Tbsp. lemon juice

4 c. onions, chopped
4 c. green peppers, chopped
8 c. tomato sauce (low salt)
4 Tbsp. basil

Combine all sauce ingredients, except basil, in large saucepan. Simmer 45-60 minutes. Add basil and simmer 30 minutes more.

The trick for cooking pasta is using lots of water. Bring 2 gallons of water to a rolling boil. Break spaghetti in half and drop it little by little into boiling water. Stir to prevent sticking and clumping. Boil uncovered for 15 to 20 minutes or less, depending on desired texture. Drain, rinse, serve. Add sauce. Garnish with lemon wedges and fresh parsley. Serve with tossed salad and low-salt, low-fat Italian dressing. Have sour-dough or whole wheat bread with garbanzo spread (see page 156).

Rice Salad (serves 6)

4 c. cooked brown rice
¼ c. mild vinegar
1 c. cooked peas or garbanzos
½ c. green onion, chopped
1 cucumber, chopped
¼ c. parsley, chopped

3 Tbsp. lemon juice
¼ tsp. dry mustard or
  1 tsp. basil
2 med. tomatoes, chopped
1 green pepper, chopped
2 stalks celery, chopped

Mix lemon juice, mustard, dill weed and vinegar. Pour over cooked rice. Toss well. Chill rice 30 minutes, then add rest of ingredients. Chill 2 hrs. before serving on bed of !ettuce leaves, garnished with tomato wedges or cherry tomatoes cut in half and watercress.

Excellent for hot summer day. Can be used for pita bread stuffing, and leftovers can be added to soups.

Lasagna With Spinach[5] (serves 10)

If you have not developed a liking for spinach yet, try this dish—you'll become a convert!

2 bunches fresh spinach (1 lb.)

1 lb. whole wheat lasagna noodles

Sauce:

1 tsp. minced garlic
½ lb. sliced mushrooms (1 cup)
2 tsp. oregano flakes
1 Tbsp. parsley flakes

2 onions, chopped (1 c.)

½ lrg. green pepper, chopped
1½ tsp. basil flakes
1 Tbsp. lemon juice

28 oz. can tomatoes with ½ the liquid in can; chop in blender 3 secs.

Filling:

2 egg whites
½ c. grated sapsago cheese (or Parmesan)

1 Tbsp. parsley flakes
½ c. buttermilk (nonfat)
3 c. lowfat cottage cheese

Preparations:

Spinach: Wash, remove stems, plunge in hot water 10 secs., chop wilted spinach fine.

Noodles: Cook (don't overcook, should be firm), drain.

Sauce: Combine all ingredients in large saucepan. Simmer about one hour.

Filling: Beat egg whites and mix with cottage cheese, then add the rest of ingredients.

Layering: Place thin sauce layer on bottom of shallow baking dish (13″ x 9″ x 2″). Place ⅓ of noodles on top, then ⅓ of filling, then ⅓ of sauce. Repeat process twice more. Top layer should be sauce. Bake for 1 hr. at 375°. Garnish with fresh parsley and lemon slices.

Rice Burgers (makes 9 patties)

1¼ c. brown cooked rice
1 Tbsp. corn flake crumbs
3/8 c. chopped walnuts
1 Tbsp. chopped green pepper
2 egg whites

2 tsp. oil
1 Tbsp. skim milk
1 Tbsp. chopped onion
1 tsp. poultry seasoning
½ tsp. salt

Mix together all ingredients and form into patties. Fry with Pam spray in electric skillet at 375° or teflon pan.

SAVORY LEGUMES

Legumes should be high on your list of food choices. They can be eaten fresh, sprouted or dried. They are abundant (there are some 30-40 varieties, if you look for them), nutritionally packed, inexpensive, simple to prepare, yet they have a delicious goodness, and their high bulk factor makes it difficult to overeat calorically. It's an important staple in any health-enhancing diet. Legumes, such as beans, lentils, peas, etc. offer: simplicity, variety, economy, exceptional nutrition (low fat, no cholesterol high fiber, plenty of minerals and vitamins, low sodium), tasty meals and they contribute to optimum health.

Legumes are the perfect food for the cook-in-a-hurry. All you have to do is dump a package of beans in a crockpot of water! The only problem with most cooks in a hurry to get dinner on the table is a lack of planning. You have to start your preparations the day before.

Cooking Beans (6 servings)

2¼ c. dry beans (1 lb.)   7 c. boiling water

Method 1:

Wash with cold water. Add beans to boiling water in large kettle (beans will expand about 2½ times, so be sure pot is large enough). Bring to a full boil. Turn off heat. Let stand one hour or more. Bring to boil again, and let gently boil until tender (simmer). Except for peas and lentils (30-45 minutes), most beans take 2 to 3 hours to simmer.

Note: There is evidence that beans cooked this way cause less flatulence (gas).

Method 2:

Soak beans overnight. Drain. Add drained beans to rapidly boiling water. Heat to boiling point. Boil until tender. Simmer until well done.

Some Tips

The *quickest* way is to cook most of the beans in a pressure cooker. After the soaking, pressure cooking takes 3 minutes (for kidney beans) to 30 minutes (soybeans).

The *most convenient* way is to cook legumes overnight in a crockpot. Dry beans and these slow cookers with their predictable temperature controls are made for each other.

When you cook beans, you may want to add one chopped onion and some chopped or whole tomatoes. Sliced carrots and chopped celery are also excellent. Add your seasoning always towards the end, about 20-30 minutes before serving.

Be adventuresome when you season beans and peas. Their delicate flavors take gratefully to a sprinkle of this, a dash of that. Onion and garlic, celery, green pepper, and herbs give special flavors.

Prepare a large batch of beans, then freeze in small containers. Heat in microwave for a quick meal. There are many uses for leftover beans, and they keep in the refrigerator at least a week.

Split Pea Soup (serves 6)

1 c. split peas	6 c. water
1 c. sauteed onions	¼ c. barley
1 bay leaf	
1 potato, chopped	1 tsp. thyme
1 carrot, chopped	⅓ c. parsley, chopped
1 celery stalk, chopped	1 tsp. sweet basil

Add peas, water, onions, barley and bay leaf to crockpot and cook until "almost" done. Add remaining ingredients and cook another 45-60 minutes. Add water if necessary.

Leftovers can be used for sandwich spread or used as potato topping.

Peggy's Family Beans[4] (serves 6)

1 lb. kidney beans	3 c. water
3 onions, chopped	2 cloves garlic, minced
8 oz. canned tomato sauce	¼ c. pitted dates
Lite salt to taste	1 c. water

Cook beans with garlic, onions and tomato sacue in crockpot until "almost" done. Liquefy dates in 1 c. water and add to beans. Let simmer for another hour. Salt to taste. Make sure beans are always covered with liquid.

These beans are even better the day after they're made. And the day after that!

Sloppy Lentils[6] (serves 6)

2 c. lentils	1 onion, chopped
1 carrot, chopped	1 green pepper, chopped
4 c. water	4 c. tomato sauce
1 Tbsp. parsley flakes	1 bay leaf
½ tsp. sweet basil	¼ tsp. garlic powder
1 Tbsp. low salt tamari	

Place lentils, onions, carrots, green pepper in crockpot. Cook until "almost" done. Add tomato sauce and seasoning and simmer for another 30 to 45 minutes.

Serve over whole wheat bread, muffins, or whole grains, like rice. Can also be used as topping for baked potato.

Black Beans over Rice[2] (serves 6)

A great bean recipe! Great colors. Serve with salad, bread and fruit for dessert—a real feast!

Beans:

1¼ c. black beans	5 c. water
1 clove garlic, minced	½ tsp. Lite salt
1 c. onion, chopped	1 green pepper, chopped
1 onion, peeled and stuck with 3 whole cloves.	

Rice:

4 c. cooked brown rice (1½ c. uncooked rice)

Salsa:

16 oz. unsalted, unpeeled tomatoes, drained	¾ c. diced red onion
1 Tbsp. mild vinegar	2 cloves garlic, minced
½ c. parsley, chopped fine	3 dashes Tabasco sauce (optional)

In small bowl, break up tomatoes with spoon. Add other ingredients, cover and refrigerate to let flavors blend.

Cook beans in crockpot until getting tender. Add garlic and clove-studded onion and Lite Salt and cook one hour more. Saute onions and green peppers. Take whole onion with cloves from beans, discard. Instead, add sauted onions and green peppers. Stir, cook a few minutes to blend flavors.

Serve black beans over cooked rice. Top with salsa.

Esau's Pottage[3] (serves 6)

⅓ c. brown rice
1 c. sauteed onions
herbs to taste (Mrs. Dash)

4 c. water
1 c. lentils

Add all ingredients to crockpot and cook until done. Add herbs shortly before serving. Slow cooking makes this delicious. Garnish with parsley, watercress and slices of red bell pepper.

Baked Beans (serves 8)

2 c. pink beans
6 c. water
1 clove garlic, minced

1 lrg. onion, chopped
3 Tbsp. parsley, minced
1 tsp. salt

Cook beans; drain and save liquid. Put onions and garlic into baking dish; add beans, salt and saved liquid until beans are covered. Bake covered at 250° 2 to 3 hrs.; uncover and add parsley for last part of baking.

Serve with some sliced green-ripe olives on top; garnish with lemon wedges. Serve with brown rice and a green salad.

Tofu "A La King" (serves 8)

2 boxes Tofu
3 cloves garlic
1 med. onion, chopped
1 tsp. onion salt
1 tsp. curry

½ tsp. turmeric
1 tsp. soy sauce
1 can mushroom soup
¼ c. yogurt or buttermilk
green onions and parsley, as
        desired

Drain tofu of its liquid. Freeze in its container to achieve firmer tofu. Thaw tofu when ready to use. Squeeze out as much liquid as possible. Steam garlic and onions in wok or teflon skillet. Preheat broiler oven to 425°. Dice tofu. Season with onion salt, turmeric and soy sauce.

Broil in oven until slightly brown. Turn once or twice. Combine browned tofu with steamed garlic and onions. Add mushroom soup, yogurt or buttermilk and curry powder. Mix well. Makes excellent scrambled egg look-a-like—only better. Add green onions and parsley and bring to a quick boil in skillet before serving. Delicious served in pita bread with crisp lettuce.

Use only occasionally, since tofu is quite rich in protein and has a fair amount of inherent fat.

SPROUTS—A NATURALLY GOOD FOOD

SPROUTS ARE DELICIOUS: Enjoy them raw . . . to spark up salads and sandwiches, as snacks, condiments, garnishes, or for complete meals.

Eat them cooked . . . in baked goods, gourmet entrees, casseroles, soups or stews.

Sprinkle a hearty helping of almost any kind of sprouts in a bowl of your favorite soup.

SPROUTS ARE NUTRITIOUS: They are nutrient-manufacturing plants! They are rich in vitamins, minerals and enzymes that multiply during sprouting and are a natural source of fiber. Dieters delight in sprouts. They are very low in calories, but rich in essential nutrients.

SPROUTS ARE ECONOMICAL: One rounded tablespoon of alfalfa seeds produces one quart of sprouted vegetables. Most varieties of seeds will yield 6-8 times their volume in sprouts—nutritious vegetables for pennies a serving.

Sprouts! Pound for pound, penny for penny, the most nutritious and economical food you can eat.

Three Easy Steps to Make Your Own Sprouts
(Growing time 3-5 days)

1. Pour measured amount of seeds and water into any standard wide mouth jar. This will usually be a ratio of 1 part seeds to 4 parts water. Place the proper screen top on the jar and soak seeds overnight.

2. The following morning, drain your soak water through the screen top. Now, rinse your sprouts. Hold under a running faucet until jar is filled. Swirl gently and drain. **Rinse sprouts every morning and evening.** Rinse more often if desired for slightly faster growth. Stand jar on screen top feet for ventilation during draining. Following draining, prop jar at an angle with screen top facing down. This will insure proper ventilation during sprouting.

3. As sprouts grow and throw off seed hulls, change to a larger screen top. Now you can rinse hulls away. Hold the jar at a slight angle under a running faucet. Swirl sprouts around as the jar fills and overflows. Hulls will be flushed out the top. Continue swirling under running water until most hulls are rinsed away. This may take two or more rinsings. Drain well. Continue rinse cycle until harvest!

SPROUT TABLE			
Seed Variety	**Dry Seed**	**Yield**	**Growing Time**
[1]Garbanzos	¾ cup	1 quart	3-5 days
Kidney Beans	1⅓ cup	1 quart	3-4 days
Lentils	¾ cup	1 quart	3-4 days
Mung Beans	⅓ cup	1 quart	3-4 days
Soybeans	1⅓ cup	1 quart	3-5 days
[2]Wheat Berries	1 cup	1 quart	3-6 days
[3]Alfalfa	2 Tbsp.	1 quart	4-5 days
Radish	¼ cup	1 quart	3-5 days
Sunflower	½ cup	1 cup	2-3 days

[1]can be eaten raw, or steamed
[2]excellent if in breadmaking
[3]ideal for eating raw in salads, as pita bread filling, and as soup topping

SCREEN TOP TIPS

Fine Screen: Rinse and drain alfalfa, cabbage, radish and other small seeds.

Medium Screen: Rinse and drain lentils, mung beans, wheat and other larger seeds. Rinse hulls away from alfalfa, cabbage and sprouts of similar size.

Coarse Screen: Rinse and drain black eye peas, garbanzo, peanuts, and other large seeds. Rinse hulls away from mung beans, radish, and sprouts of similar size.

Some More Tips

• For all seeds, soak water should be warm and rinse water should be tepid. Final rinse water should be cold. Ideal sprouting temperature is 65-75 degrees.

• The soak water from most seeds is full of valuable nutrients. You can use it for making soups, teas, or even watering your plants. Do not drink or use soybean soak water.

• Avoid growing sprouts in direct sunlight.

• Seed hulls are not harmful and contain nutritional value, but most people prefer removing them to minimize mold problems and insure the freshest tasting sprouts.

• Stored sprouts must be kept cold. Store jar covered with fine screen top in refrigerator. To freshen stored sprouts, use screen top and rinse with cold water and drain well.

• You can prop your jar of sprouts almost anywhere for ventilation during sprouting. Prop jar with screen top facing down in a dish drain, in a deep bowl, or just propped up on a counter.

SOUPS AND VEGETABLES

Soups, prepared in a crockpot, are ideal for cooks who have to serve meals-in-a-hurry. A good "hefty" soup plus some sandwiches make an excellent combination for a meal, which can be augmented by a salad of cucumbers and tomatoes (or tossed salad) and topped off with some fresh fruit as dessert.

Crunchy cabbage, crisp celery, cooked carrots and bright banana squash all bring sunshine to the table and the sparkle of health to the family. Deep yellow-orange and dark green leafy vegetables particularly contain an abundance of important nutrients.

The trick for the cook is to prepare the vegetables in a way to make them look beautiful and appetizing, to keep their color, texture and flavor—all with maximum retention of their food values. To accomplish this, just follow the 3 R's:

1. Reduce the amount of water used (waterless cookware and microwaving is ideal)
2. Reduce the length of cooking time
3. Reduce the amount of surface area exposed

Always add vegetable to water that's already boiling. Many vegetables (such as broccoli flowerets) will thus be steamed within 3 to 5 minutes. Cook in covered pan. Do not remove cover while cooking, or stir them. Cook vegetables whole, or in large piece when possible. Also, try to break the habit of adding salt to the water. Some "Mrs. Dash" (salt free, low pepper) seasoning or other herbs, (see page 201) can be added with the vegetables into the boiling water in the shallow pan.

Overcooking of vegetables causes some nutrient loss and adversely affects the color, flavor, and texture. It may become necessary to reeducate your and your family's taste to enjoy crispy cooked vegetables, oriental style. Give it some time, and you'll wonder how you could have ever eaten those mushy, limp, nutrition-eroded and anemic looking vegetables.

Vegetable Platter Combinations

- Cauliflower in the center, small whole beets on the outside, or green beans and carrots.
- Mound of whole baby carrots surrounded by green peas and small steamed onions.
- Mound of cooked broccoli surrounded by yellow gooseneck zucchini (diagonally sliced) and crisp carrot sticks. Arrange mounds of raw grated beets, carrots, turnips. You may add kidney beans, garbanzos, or pea pods to such a display platter.

Broccoli-Cauliflower Duo (serves 6)

3 c. bite-sized broccoli flowerets plus pinch of tarragon
½ c. boiling water in shallow pan
3 c. bite-sized cauliflowerets plus pinch of rosemary and 3 Tbsp. lemon juice
½ c. boiling water in shallow pan

Simmer broccoli with tarragon until crispy-tender and still bright green.

Simmer cauliflower with rosemary and lemon juice (to keep cauliflower white) until crispy-tender. Add a sprinkle of red paprika powder for accent.

Toss, or serve separately—hot or cold.

Cabbage Crepes[1] (2 cups, serves 8)

Crepes (see page 134)
Filling:

2 c. finely chopped, sauteed onions	4 c. shredded cabbage
¾ c. skim milk	1 tsp. caraway seed or dill weed
1 tsp. Lite Salt	2 Tbsp. whole wheat flour

To sauteed onions add cabbage and caraway seeds; cover and steam, stirring occasionally until cabbage is tender. Combine remaining ingredients and pour over cabbage. Simmer 3 to 4 minutes until thickened. Fill each crepe with ¼ c. of filling, roll up crepe or fold over.

Serve at once. To serve later, put into baking dish, cover and bake at 300° for 20 minutes.

Baked Acorn Squash (serves 6)

3 acorn squash
12 oz. can crushed pineapple
¼ tsp. ground ginger

3 carrots, grated
3 Tbsp. raisins

Cut squash in half; remove seeds. Place squash in baking pan. Mix remaining ingredients and spoon it into squash shells. Bake at 350° for 40 minutes.

Baked Carrots (serves 6)

1 lb. carrots, sliced
2 Tbsp. dried parsley flakes
¼ c. boiling water

½ c. finely sliced onions
½ tsp. Lite Salt

Place alternate layers of carrots and onions with seasoning into a casserole. Have 4-6 layers. Pour water over all. Cover. Bake at 375° until tender.

Vegetable Bean Soup

1 c. navy beans
5 c. water
¾ c. celery, chopped
1 tsp. "Mrs. Dash"

½ c. barley
¾ c. onion, sliced
1 c. carrots
1 tsp. Lite Salt

Soak beans and barley overnight. Place in crockpot. Add seasoning 45 minutes before it's done.

Quick Garbanzo Soup (serves 6, 2 cups each)

3 green onions, chopped
1 onion, chopped
32 oz. garbanzos, drained
2 carrots, sliced
some parsley, finely chopped
6 oz. tomato paste (unsalted)
5 c. water

1 clove garlic, minced
2 c. celery, chopped
1 c. potato, diced
1 green pepper, chopped
¼ tsp. "Mrs. Dash" seasoning
1 tsp. McKay's Chicken-Style
    seasoning

Saute white onion, garlic, celery. Add remaining ingredients. Bring to boil; simmer for 20 minutes. Stir well before serving.

Easy Lentil Soup (serves 6, 2 cups each)

2½ c. lentils
4 green onions, chopped
1 c. celery, chopped
1 bay leaf
½ tsp. McKay's Chicken-style seasoning

10 c. water
1 c. carrots, chopped
1½ c. potatoes, diced
½ tsp. "Mrs. Dash" seasoning

Put everything in crockpot overnight. Before serving add tablespoon of lemon juice.

Zucchini Soup (serves 6)

6 c. zucchini, cubed
2 c. potatoes, unpeeled, chunked
1 c. onion, chopped
1 lrg. garlic clove, quartered
3 tsps. chicken-style flavoring
2 c. water
¼ c. chives (reserved for garnish)

½ tsp. "Mrs. Dash" seasoning
1 c. dry skim milk
1 tsp. Lite Salt
½ tsp. basil, crushed
½ tsp. dill
¼ tsp. paprika

Place zucchini, potatoes, onion, and garlic in a soup kettle.

Dissolve chicken-style flavoring in two cups water and pour over the vegetables. Cover and cook 8 to 10 minutes or until the vegetables are tender.

Puree the cooked vegetables, liquid stock, dry milk and herbs in a blender until smooth.

Return to soup kettle and heat until hot enough to serve. Pour into bowls and garnish with chives.

Spanish Gazpacho Soup (serves 4)

2 c. tomatoes, chopped
½ c. celery, chopped
1 c. cucumber, peeled & chopped
¼ c. green pepper, chopped
1 c. canned green chili salsa
Garnish: lime slices

1 c. zucchini, chopped
4 c. tomato juice
½ c. green onions, chopped
1 clove garlic, minced
Lime juice to taste

Combine chopped tomatoes, zucchini, celery in a bowl and mix together. Transfer ⅓ of this mixture to a blender, add some of the tomato juice, and puree. Pour the pureed vegetables back into the bowl and mix in the remaining ingredients. Chill. Serve garnished with lime slices.

Cheese-Onion Soup (serves 8)

10 lrg. onions, thinly sliced	12 c. water
2 bay leaves	½ tsp. "Mrs. Dash"
4 Tbsp. unbleached all-purpose flour	8 sliced sourdough toast
	8 Tbsp. grated fresh sapsago cheese

Place 1 sliced onion in a small baking pan and set aside. Place the remaining onions in a large saucepan with the water, bay leaves, and "Mrs. Dash." Cover and cook this until the onions are tender. Remove the bay leaves. Sprinkle the flour over the onion slices in a baking pan; put it under the broiler until the flour has browned and some of the onions have burned. Add a little water and stir until smooth. Add a small amount of the soup, stirring until smooth, then return all to the soup. Heat the soup, stirring constantly until boiling and slightly thickened. Pour the soup into 4 individual crocks, and trim the toast to fit on top of each. Sprinkle the toast with grated cheese. Put it under the broiler until the cheese melts. Serve at once.

Easy Zucchini[7] (serves 6)

6 small zucchinis	3 c. tomato juice
1½ tsp. thyme	½ tsp. "Mrs. Dash" seasoning

Slice zucchini into ¼ inch thick slices. Place them into baking dish with other ingredients. Cover and bake at 375° for 20 minutes.

Variation:

4 c. zucchini	2 tomatoes, sliced
1 c. cottage cheese	1½ tsp. thyme
½ tsp. "Mrs. Dash"	1 onion, sliced

Put half of zucchini in baking dish. Add layer of **half** of tomatoes, onions and cottage cheese. Mix thyme and "Mrs. Dash," sprinkle half of it over top. Repeat layer. Bake at 375° for 35 minutes. Garnish with parsley.

Barley-Tomato Vegetable Soup (serves 8)

1 c. barley	1 c. peas
1 c. onion, chopped	1 c. celery, chopped
1 c. carrots, chopped	½ c. green pepper, chopped
1 c. white cabbage, shredded	1 c. potato, diced
½ c. frozen "mixed" vegetables	7 c. water
1 c. canned tomato juice	1 c. canned diced tomatoes
2 Tbsp. lemon juice	¼ tsp. marjoram
¼ tsp. basil	½ tsp. onion powder
½ tsp. garlic powder	½ tsp. dried parsley

Microwave overnight-soaked barley for 20 minutes. Then add all ingredients except seasonings to crockpot. Simmer. When "almost" done, add seasoning and simmer for another 30 minutes. Add chopped parsley just before serving.

SALADS AND FRUITS

Capture the beauty, the vitality, and the abundance nature provides in salads. Your can eat with your eyes and enjoy the taste.

General Guidelines for Salad

- Contrast texture, color, form, flavor in tossed salads
- Break with hand (bitesize)
- Chill salad (preferably on ice)
- Use chilled plates/bowls
- Have different dressings available with **small** ladling spoons
- Garnish salad bowls with lemon wedges, yellow squash slices, etc.

Banana Popsicles

Peel and cut banana crosswise in half. Insert an ice cream stick through the length of it. Dip the banana in skim milk and then in Grape Nut "crumbs" that have been flavored with a dash of cinnamon or nutmeg. Freeze.

Fruit in Season

Watermelon or honeydew melon, strawberries, cantaloupe, etc., washed and chilled.

California Lettuce Salad[1] (serves 12)

1 lrg. head butter lettuce torn
into bitesize pieces
2 lrg. tomatoes, chopped
⅓ avocado, cubed (½ cup)
½ c. watercress sprouts

1 cucumber (peeling removed),
thinly sliced
½ c. purple onion, chopped
4 Tbsp. parsley, chopped

Bean Salad[2] (serves 10)

Drain and combine:
16 oz. can kidney beans
16 oz. can garbanzos

16 oz. can pinto beans
16 oz. can corn

Then add and toss:
½ c. green onion, chopped
¾ c. celery, chopped

½ c. parsley, chopped
4 oz. can diced green chilis

Dressing: use commercially available lowfat, low salt dressings; or use Italian dressing.

Citrus Salad Dressing[1]

¼ tsp. paprika
¼ tsp. salad herbs
3 Tbsp. frozen orange juice
concentrate, undiluted

¼ tsp. dill weed
½ tsp. garlic salt
2½ tsp. lemon juice

Makes 4 tablespoons. (24 calories per tablespoon)

Italian Dressing[7]

¼ c. lemon juice
¼ c. unsweetened apple juice
½ tsp. dry mustard
½ tsp. garlic powder
1/8 tsp thyme

¼ c. mild vinegar
½ tsp. oregano
½ tsp. onion powder
½ tsp. patrika
1/8 tsp. rosemary

Combine all ingredients in blender. Blend well. Chill and refrigerate (at least 2 days to permit flavors to "marry")

Makes ¾ cup. (5 calories per tablespoon)

Salsa #1[7] (1 cup)

2 medium tomatoes
4 fresh serrano chilies
8 sprigs corriander
½ c. cold water

2 onions
1 clove garlic, minced
1 tsp. lemon juice

Blenderize—that's all!

Salsa #2[7]

1 16 oz. can whole tomatoes
undrained and chopped
1 ripe tomato, peeled & chopped
½ onion, finely chopped
¼ tsp. basil

½ green pepper, finely chopped
1 Tbsp. diced canned green chilis
½ Tbsp. mild vinegar
¼ tsp. oregano

Combine all the ingredients, stirring well. Use the Salsa as a dip, relish, salad dressing or a baked potato topping.

Serves 4, or more if used for a dip.

Thousand Island Dressing[7]

1 c. Mock Sour Cream (page 157)
1 Tbsp. tomato paste
2 Tbsp. green pepper, chopped

1 Tbsp. onion, chopped
¼ tsp. garlic powder
¼ tsp. "Mrs. Dash" seasoning

Combine all the ingredients and mix well. Thin the dressing with skim milk, if necessary. Refrigerate it until ready to use. Makes 1¼ cups.

Cauliflower Salad (serves 10)

1 head cauliflowerets
1 green pepper, chopped
1 c. lowfat yogurt
Pinch of "Mrs. Dash"

1 2-oz. can black olives, sliced
1 clove garlic, minced
2 Tbsp. lemon juice

Toss green pepper and cauliflowerets and olives. Combine seasoning and yogurt in blender. Pour over vegetables and stir.

Tossed Salad (serves 12)

1½ heads bronze leaf or butter lettuce
10 leaves of French sorrel
½ c. radish sprouts
3 tomatoes (8 wedges each)

1½ c. watercress leaves
¾ c. parsley
1 c. alfalfa sprouts
1½ c. croutons (from whole wheat bread)

Carrot-Raisin Salad² (serves 6)

4½ c. shredded carrots
¾ c. plain lowfat yogurt

1 c. raisins
¼ c. cottage cheese

Blend yogurt and cottage cheese. Then combine with raisins and carrots. Some fennel or anise seeds will give a special accent. Garnish with slice of pineapple.

Zestful Lemon-Dill Dressing (2 cups)

2 c. lowfat cottage cheese
2 Tbsp. lemon juice
½ tsp. lemon peel, grated

2 tsp. dill weed
1 tsp. celery seed, crushed
4 Tbsp. skim milk

Blenderize. Chill. Excellent on salad greens or cooked vegetables such as zucchini or broccoli.

Ambrosia Fruit Cup

Fresh fruit (whatever is available; apples, pears, bananas, berries, grapes, melon, papaya, pineapple, etc.)

Mock sour cream (see page 157)

Frozen apple juice concentrate

Grated lemon rind (peel and use side of rind next to fruit to avoid paraffin, coloring, etc.)

Cut assorted fruits into bitesized cubes and place in individual serving dishes. Make topping of mock sour cream flavored with a little frozen apple juice concentrate and grated lemon rind. (Fruit cups may be made up in advance and refrigerated one hour or more, or served unchilled.)

Kadota Figs and Grapes (serves 6)

1 lb. canned kadota figs, water packed
1 c. white seedless grapes

Combine figs and grapes in a small compote dish. Add ice cubes to chill and serve.

Papaya Split[1] (serves 12)

3 chilled ripe papaya, halved lengthwise and seeded
3 c. honeydew melon balls
3 c. frozen unsweetened blueberries
2 tsp. lime juice

Place papaya on lettuce leaf. Sprinkle honeydew and blueberries with lime juice; put into papaya halves. Fruits should all be chilled prior to use.

Gourmet Salad Dressing (serves 12)

1 c. plain yogurt
1 Tbsp. lemon juice
1 clove garlic, minced

½ tsp. dill weed or fresh dill
¼ onion, chopped

Blenderize quickly. Chill for one hour for flavors to blend.

Stuffed Baked Apples[1] (serves 6)

6 large Rome Beauty apples, Golden Delicious, or other baking apples
3 tsp. raisins
¼ c. honey
1 tsp. vanilla extract

3 tsp. walnuts, chopped
1 tsp. coriander (ground)
1 tsp. lemon juice

Water to cover bottom of baking pan ¼ inch deep

Wash and core apples from stem side without piercing the "bottom" of apples. Place in deep baking pan. Mix raisins and walnuts; put a teaspoon of mixture in center of each apple.

Mix honey, coriander, lemon juice, vanilla; pour a teaspoonfull into center of each apple.

Mix a cup of water with rest of honey mixture; pour over apples in baking pan; pour more water around apples to make ¼ inch deep; cover with lid or foil. Bake at 350° until tender when pierced with fork (about 45 minutes). Serve hot and plain.

Diehl-ight Banana Ice Cream

Freeze six peeled bananas (at least 24 hours). Blend in osterizer with a half cup of water. Add 2 tsp. vanilla or almond extract. Add 2 tsp. lemon or orange juice. The addition of ice cubes will further thicken the ice cream. For a change in flavor, add 1 cup of pineapple chunks and blend thoroughly. Garnish with mint leaf and serve with a clear conscience.

Banana Split Lite

1 banana, split lengthwise
Fruits in season, such as,

½ c. blueberries
½ c. cantaloupe "balls"
½ c. sliced seedless grapes
½ c. mandarin orange segments
½ c. cassava/honeydew "balls"
1 c. pineapple chunks

Place banana halves on bottom of serving dish. Add fruits in season, except for the pineapple. Thicken pineapple with some cornstarch or tapioca. Bring to a quick boil. Stir in some coconut flakes. Let cool and pour over the banana-fruit mixture. Garnish with a few walnut halves and a mint leaf. Chill before serving.

Fruit Soup (serves 6)

3½ c. unsweetened pineapple
    juice
1½ c. seedless grapes, sliced
3 bananas, sliced
3½ Tbsp. Minute Tapioca
2 small apples, diced
2 cans peaches, diced
3 c. strawberries or raspberries,
    sliced

Soak tapioca for five minutes in pineapple juice. Then cook juice and tapioca until thick. Add the fruits. Serve warm or better yet: chill! Garnish by slicing some of banana over top and add a mint leaf.

Oriental Lychees With Pineapple (serves 8)

1 lb. (drained weight) of lychees in light syrup (or water packed)
1 quart-size can pineapple chunks (fresh or water-packed)
Some frozen cranberries for garnish

Combine fruits, add ice cubes, and garnish with mint leaf in a small compote bowl.

AND SOME MORE . . .

Mock Cheese Cake (serves 8)

1 c. plain yogurt
1 c. cottage cheese, lowfat
1 c. strawberries

1 apple, grated
1 banana

Blenderize quickly yogurt and cottage cheese. Mash and mix fruits and combine with blenderized mixture. Fill in 9″ graham cracker crust pie shell. Freeze. Garnish and serve with a clear conscience.

Garbanzo Spread

1 can garbanzos, drained
½ tsp. onion powder
½ tsp. butter salt (optional)

2 Tbsp. lemon juice
¼ tsp. garlic powder
Pinch of herbs, as desired

Blenderize, adding just enough garbanzo juice to produce smooth spread.

Bean Spread

2 c. cooked beans, drained
6 Tbsp. tomato sauce
¼ tsp. onion powder

1/8 tsp. sweet basil
1/8 tsp. garlic powder

Blend beans until smooth, adding bean liquid to make a thick puree. Pour puree into top of double boiler. Add remaining ingredients. (Grind the herbs into a powder before adding.) Cook until the mixture is thoroughly heated, stirring frequently. Chill.

Multi-Purpose Sauce (serves 6)

4 tomatoes, diced
1½ stems celery, minced

1 large onion, chopped
Dash of paprika or cummin
and ½ tsp. "Mrs. Dash"

Cook until tender. Blenderize.

Mock Sour Cream[7]

Skim milk   Hoop cheese (or dry curd cheese)
Lemon juice to taste

Pour 1 cup milk into blender. Add handful of hoop cheese; blend. Stop blender and stir. Add more liquid or more cheese, blending and occasionally stirring until mixture resembles sour cream in smoothness and consistency and desired volume is obtained. Vinegar or lemon juice may be added to give "sour cream" tang. For *sweet* topping add several teaspoons frozen apple juice concentrate. Fresh bananas can be blended in for sweetness and smoothness, adding nutmeg and/or cinnamon. Mock sour cream keeps well in tightly sealed plastic containers, but has tendency to thicken on standing. To thin, merely stir in a little more milk to bring back the desired consistency. Can also be frozen, then stirred vigorously after thawing.

Oven-Roasted Potatoes (12 servings)

6 potatoes   1 onion, chopped
2 tbsp. soy sauce (Kikkoman,   1 tsp. dried parsley
     milder salt-reduced brand)   1 tsp. paprika

Peel potatoes, wash and slice once in half lengthwise. Cut potatoes into ¼ inch thick slices and line them up in a teflon baking pan. Sprinkle with onion, parsley, paprika, and soy sauce. Bake (broil) at 400° until brown and puffed up, then turn over with spatula.

Grape Spread

½ c. Concord grape juice   1 Tbsp. Minute tapioca
1 c. currants

Heat until warm and let stand ½ hour. Simmer for about 7-10 minutes. Cover and let stand until cool. Place in container and let set overnight to hydrate the currants. Refrigerate.

Popcorn

Use a mesh hand-held popper that does not come in contact with the heat. Shake vigorously as it is popping to prevent burning.

Pineapple Suckers

Cut fresh pineapple into spears or use canned pineapple spears. Spear with flat or round wooden sticks. Roll in finely crushed macaroon coconut (unsweetened). Place in deep freeze. They may be rolled in parchment or cellophane paper. Or you may stand them up in a freezer container.

Baked Apples

6 baking apples, cored
6 Tbsp. apple juice concentrate
¼ tsp. ground cloves
½ tsp. ground cinnamon

Preheat oven to 350°. Place 1 tablespoon apple juice concentrate, mixed with cloves and cinnamon, in the center of each apple. Arrange the apples in a baking dish and add water to a depth of ½ inch. Bake, basting frequently, for ½ hour.

Dried Fruit Jam

Soak equal amounts of 2 or 3 dried fruits in unsweetened pineapple juice overnight in the refrigerator. Good combinations consist of apricots, pears or apples and dates. Place soaked fruit in blender and add enough pineapple juice to give the desired consistency. Store in refrigerator.

Crisped Tortilla Chips

1 pkg. of 12 corn tortillas
½ tsp. garlic powder (optional)
½ tsp. onion powder (optional)

Arrange the tortillas in a stack. Cut all 12 in half at once, and then into quarters. Lay these wedges on a nonstick baking sheet, avoiding overlapping. Sprinkle them with onion and garlic powder, if desired. Bake in a preheated 375-400° oven until the chips are crisp, stirring and turning to brown evenly. Remove the wedges as they are done.

HOW TO EAT OUT! *

Restaurant selection

Vegetarian restaurants are a good bet; so are healthfood restaurants. You may, of course, already have a convert in the owner and then your problems will be minimal.

Among **American** restaurants, one featuring a salad bar can be a lifesaver.

Cafeterias have the advantage of showing you exactly what you're getting before items are delivered to your table. The problem is, almost everything they serve is swimming in fats and sugars, leaving you with slim pickings.

Chinese restaurants are good because their food is customarily cooked to order. You can often get the chef to prepare a dish of steamed vegetables. Be sure to ask them to hold the MSG, sugar, oil and salt. A little dash of soy sauce goes a long way toward flavoring your food.

Italian restaurants' pasta isn't as good as the wholewheat variety you've stocked in your kitchen, but it'll do. Order unbuttered spaghetti with a tomato sauce, a cup of minestrone if it's not the fatty kind, and a dry salad dressed with lemon juice, or mild vinegar. Remembering to avoid parmesan, and restrict those salty olives.

Seafood restaurants are OK, if you want to eat fish. Stay away from the high-cholesterol shellfish and butter and tartar sauce. Have your seafood choice prepared without fats—broiled, baked, or poached (not fried).

Things to remember before you leave for "eating out":

• Don't get into the habit of eating out too often. It can get wearying to make a production of ordering your foods in the enemy camp.

• Eat something to take the edge off your appetite before you leave home. This will minimize the seductive power of an unfriendly menu.

• Restaurants appreciate being called in advance for special requests. This courtesy improves your chances of getting what you want.

• When it comes right down to the nitty-gritty, it's your strength of character that will determine whether the restaurateur is going to serve you—or you're sheepishly going to take what is served everybody else.

• Remember that a good restaurateur enjoys making you happy. He survives on repeat business.

• Steer clear of cheap restaurants. Usually the prices aren't that much lower—but the food is. Cheap restaurants pack their dishes with fat and sweets to compensate for the lack of real food.

• Beware of hospital restaurants. Paradoxically, they are among the worst for fatty, cholesterol-laden, sugary foods.

• If you're too easily corrupted by gastronomic allurements, join your friends at the restaurant after dinner for socializing.

Things to remember when ordering

• Don't nod "yes" when you're asked if you want sour cream with your baked potato. Try it just with chives or cottage cheese.

• You can spice the blandness of your hardy baked potato with a nonoil salsa. West Coast restaurants are more likely to have salsa on hand than others.

• Ask for sourdough rolls or bread immediately. If they don't have them, eat the rolls they do have.

• If there are only one or two dishes that won't throw you off your diet, don't hesitate to load up on them and forget the rest. You may feel cheated eating nothing but salad and soup and (occasionally) having to pay for a noneaten entree may be wiser than having eaten it. Just remember that less is more!

• Sometimes the only acceptable vegetable is a baked potato—since most restaurants smother vegetables in butter or margarine. In that case, eat two baked potatoes.

• If you eat at one restaurant regularly, let the owner look over your diet and favorite recipes. If he wants to keep your business, usually he'll manage to include several of them among his repertoire.

• In vegetarian restaurants, don't forget to defend yourself against their oils, cheeses, nuts, avocado, honey, etc.

• In salad bars, stay away from marinated vegetables (too much oil). Load up on red onions, bamboo shoots, garbanzo beans (chickpeas), raw cauliflower, broccoli, celery, radishes, etc. Avoid croutons, cheese toppings, cole slaw, grated eggs, and the like.

• You can survive in a Mexican restaurant by ordering a pile of warm corn tortillas (careful that you're not getting an omelette!) and getting the chef to customblend a taco or enchilada without cheese. You can complement these with a lettuce and tomato salad—possible on top of your enchilada or inside your taco.

• Make your baked potato order a restaurant habit. If you don't three guesses what you're going to find alongside your entree.

Breakfast Ideas

• Hot oatmeal or Cream of Wheat, Shredded Wheat or Grape Nuts.

• Ask for nonfat milk.

• Order a grapefruit half, a sliced orange, melon, berries, or sliced banana.

• Ask for dry toast or rolls and a pot of hot water with lemon slice.

Lunch and Dinner Ideas

• Don't fret over occasional deviations in a restaurant. But if you visit a restaurant regularly, be very strict.

• A great standby: a large green salad without dressing (lemon juice) or with a prudent amount of low calorie dressing (but watch out for the salt!)

• Standby dessert: any fresh fruit.

• Standby appetizers: split pea, navy bean, lentil, or vegetable soups (if made without all that fat).

• Fresh or steamed vegetables—without butter—are ideal. Try artichokes, mushrooms, zucchini, corn on the cob, green beans or peas, and baked potatoes.

---

* Excerpted from *The Pritikin Program* by N. Pritikin and P. M. McGrady, Grosset & Dunlap, Inc., 1979.

1

The Silent Disease

LaVerne: We are excited having Drs. Hans and Lily Diehl and their children, Byron and Carmen, with us. I know that this will be a special program.

Now, Dr. Hans, in talking about high blood pressure, you referred to it as the "silent killer." How about the "silent disease," as some refer to the breakdown in family communication? Is that quite prevalent in our society today?

Dr. Hans: I'm afraid that could be right. All too many families live lives of quiet desperation—overcome by social pressures, work obligations, children's crazy schedules, and part-time jobs. Consequently, we eat on the run. We grab as we can. And meals are seldom eaten together anymore, and if we do eat a meal together, then it's usually in a horseshoe arrangement—we are sitting around the television set with food on our TV trays.

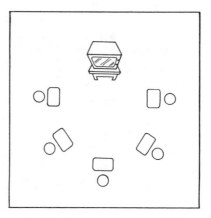

FIG. 1.1: The Horseshoe Eating Arrangement with TV at center stage.

Dr. Hans: All this then only seems to increase our emotional isolation and contributes to an erosion and breakdown of in-family communications.

LaVerne: I learned that your family recently received the "Family of the Year Award," which reads,

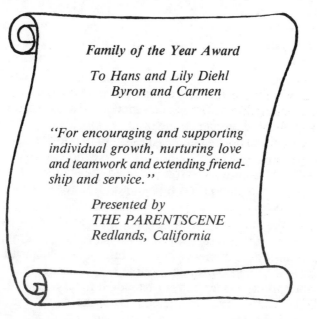

Family of the Year Award

To Hans and Lily Diehl
Byron and Carmen

"For encouraging and supporting individual growth, nurturing love and teamwork and extending friendship and service."

Presented by
THE PARENTSCENE
Redlands, California

You obviously seem to have some insights and some keys of how to work and live and love as a family. How about sharing with us your ideas on how to improve family communications?

Tell us, Hans, what have you and Lily done to keep family life alive? What are some of the basics?

Dr. Hans: Basically we have always viewed our children, Byron and Carmen, as our number *one* priority, and *then* our jobs, etc. Children need love and discipline, especially during those first six to eight years of life. After that they increasingly need independence and autonomy.

LaVerne: Lily, how do you share that love with your kids?

Dr. Lily: It's by being ourselves, doing things together and just being supportive. We have regular playnights with Scrabble, Chinese checkers, table tennis–or simply inventing pantomime charades where the children may portray some Bible characters and we have to identify them—and we only get three tries! Then the game is turned around: we do the pantomime. And guess who wins? The kids!

Or we take them shopping to teach them comparative pricing, or we expose them to reading nutrition labels at a supermarket, thus drawing them into our adult circle.

We also involve them in our professional activities whenever possible. We travel together. We concertize together. Byron is now eleven years old; Carmen is turning ten. They are emerging quite nicely as musicians, both with their violins and the piano. And it's such a joy to see them contribute musically. When Hans keynoted a national medical convention, Byron provided the entertainment on his violin and piano for a special reception for international scientists.

Dr. Hans: As a reward, I arranged to take him mountain climbing for several days with backpacks and all, an unforgettable experience both emotionally and spiritually. When Carmen spent a couple of months with her grandparents in Germany, we made it a habit to write her regularly. When Carmen came back, she made it a point to show us that we had actually sent her 24 cards and letters.

Also she was most appreciative about our regular phone calls. Obviously, since we feel emotional support for children is very important and essential, that's the very least we could have done. And yet she hardly missed us! You wouldn't believe this, but it took her five weeks before she finally told us on the phone that she missed us. To wait that long before hearing that we were missed almost "killed" us!

Whenever the children have a recital or a gymnastics performance, we make every effort to be present even to the point that I will reschedule an appointment. We want to let them know that they are important to us. And afterward we may celebrate, like going to a friend's home to watch "Herbie, the Lovebug!"

LaVerne: Byron, does your dad do something special that makes your mom happy?

Byron: O Yes! Every Friday afternoon he brings special flowers home, and I give them to her, and I say to her, "That's from your lover!" But one time when I gave her the flowers and told her that they were from her lover, she was teaching some students, and they all looked kind of shocked, until Mommy explained it to them. So I don't say that anymore when students are around.

Then on Friday night we usually have candlelight dinner, and my dad does the dishes afterwards. Well, he doesn't *always* do it. Sometimes he only has good intentions . . .

"We make every effort to be present, even if we have to reschedule an appointment."

LaVerne: But Byron, tell me, what do you do to let your mom know you love her?

Byron: I took her and Dad out on Mother's Day to play minigolf. We even let her win one game! And I always love to thank her for the good meals she cooks. We all thank her after almost every meal, especially if it is good!

LaVerne: Lily, aside from that Friday flower bouquet, do you do anything special for each other?

Dr. Lily: I try to have the house orderly when Hans comes home so that he can prepare the evening meal! Actually, I usually teach in my music studio from three to eight p.m. That means the family has to take care of themselves at suppertime. Of course I do some of those special feminine things like slipping a love note in his attache case just to keep him alert! And we both listen to each other intently, especially on the emotional level. And we help each other in projects. We are both quite affectionate. Hans is my best friend and confidante. With him I can be totally myself.

Alma: Do you have any magic in how you discipline Byron and Carmen?

Dr. Hans: Not really. We try to affirm and praise our children for anything positive and unselfish they do. This affirmation then reinforces the positive acts, and because of the positive response (strokes) they are more likely to do them again. Of course this then sets up a positive behavior and habit pattern, which through continued affirmation

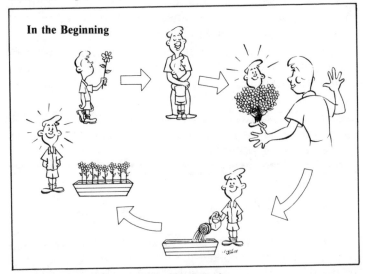

FIG. 1.2: The Positive Way to Positive Behavior
Behavior is shaped by affirming acts which lead to habits and to greater self-care.

leads to greater self-care. This in turn provides for a sense of emerging autonomy with its inherent rewards (and disappointments), which can lead to greater awareness and reality and can give a greater sense of accomplishment and self-worth. Of course the better children feel about themselves, coupled with a sense of appropriate reality, the less discipline they require. (See Fig. 1.2.)

When discipline is necessary, we try to apply it with consistency and with cool temper. The rules are few, but we enforce them. For instance, dishonesty is totally unacceptable. If they break something and tell us, there is no punishment save financial restitution. When Byron was six, he played one morning with his soccer ball in front of the glass window. I warned him about the obvious dangers and left for my office. When I cam home that night, I saw a boy with a sheepish, sad face greeting me at the door. "I need to show you something," he said with some trepidation, pointing at the cracked window pane. "But I'll pay for it!"

What Byron didn't expect was my reaction: I hugged him, put him on my arm, praised him for his honesty and courage in telling Dadddy. He couldn't believe it! He may have thought for a moment that his misdeed was rewarded! But he had learned that it was safe to admit a mistake. There was only one more thing to do: to get to his piggybank and pay for the window!

Dr. Lily: We have also used goal charts very effectively over the years. Here we negotiate with the children the goals they want to set for the next two to four weeks and what they want to do to reach them. This gives them a certain self-structure. The absence of a television set in our home simplifies rearing children, we believe. In addition to giving them points for reinforcing good behavior on their goal chart, which they tally every night, we may subtract points for poor citizenship, for example, when Byron puts down Carmen.

LaVerne: A recent survey among churchgoing people pointed out that only eight per cent of the fathers lead out in some form of family meditation on a regular basis. Do you have any suggestions?

Dr. Hans: That's a vulnerable spot for most fathers. I, too, have struggled with that, and I believe that *our day is made or broken before the kids get out of bed, when we have our personal devotional time.* Lily and I wake up around six o'clock. That gives us thirty minutes before the

---

"The relationship to our children will be more eloquent than what we could say about God."

---

youngsters take me for our half-hour of jogging. When we get back, the table is all set, we get into the showers, get dressed and we can hardly wait to have that hot seven-grain cereal with some fresh fruits. After we've had the children's short devotional lesson, we are ready to go! Secure in God's love, we have a sense of inner confidence and adequacy. We think that ultimately our relationship to them will be more eloquent than what we could say about God.

At night we make it a habit to tuck them in, but not without a bedtime story and a discussion of things that need to be cleared up or taken care of.

Lily and I feel that the time and the quality of time tell the children how much they are valued. And for the children the knowledge of being loved is worth more than gold.

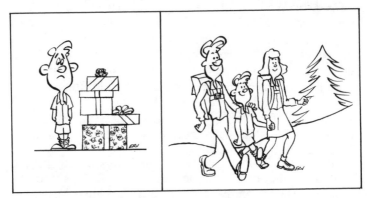

FIG. 1.3: *Presents* vs. *Presence*
"Children don't need many presents. But they do need our presence."

Friends sometimes ask us, "But how do you find the time?" We don't. We *make* the time. We set priorities and follow through as best we can. Of course it take stime to give children top priority. It's easier to give **presents.** But love cannot be found in things. Children don't need many presents; but they *do* need our **presence.** What richer contribution could anybody give to another life than to nourish a sense of self-worth, encourage self-discipline, and insure a deep internal sense of security?

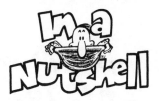

La Verne: Friend, let's summarize what some families have found helpful in keeping family life alive and in improving family communications so that the members do not fall prey to the "Silent Disease":

1. Set priorities in favor of the family.
2. Share your love with your children by
   —being yourself
   —doing things together actively
   —being supportive.
3. Make time to do thoughtful things:
   —to play together
   —to listen to each other, even on the emotional level
   —to remember that children don't need presents, but they need our presence!
4. Discipline: have few rules but enforce those few.
5. Set goals and monitor them. Goal charts can be excellent in that they provide self-structure.
6. Have a personal and family devotional life. A family that prays together stays together.

2

The Brain: Overfed And Undernourished

LaVerne: Americans consume a diet that has lost its balance. Imagine, more than *fifty per cent* of our daily calories are empty, refined calories almost totally devoid of any nutritional content!

Dr. Hans: Unfortunately many don't realize how many of these concentrated calories are well hidden, especially the fat-calories. Did you know that a three-piece chicken dinner, extra crispy, has the equivalent of eighteen pats of butter, or 650 calories from fat alone? Did you know that two handfuls of nuts have more than 1000 calories? And a banana split has, in addition to fat, more than 25 teaspoons of sugar!

LaVerne: No wonder millions are fighting the battle of the bulge!

Dr. Hans: Yes. Tragically, in our search for exotic and quick weight loss schemes we have overlooked the success principle of eating *more* natural foods, rich in fiber and nutrition, low in calories and price, and eating *less* of animal products and of refined, engineered foods.

The result is this: in the midst of plenty of calories many are starving nutritionally. Many of us are actually *overfed* and *undernourished*.

LaVerne: Let me take off on this in looking at our informational overload. Everywhere we turn we are bombarded with information: the newspaper headlines scream at us, radio and TV give us the latest information on violence, greed, stocks and bonds, and commissions release their reports. We are barraged by information, as we all know.

Now we usually think about our physical body being overfed and undernourished. But is it possible that this principle could apply to our personalities? Could it be that our computerized information has led to an overfeeding on facts and figures at the expense of building positive, ethical values and noble character so as to provide a more balanced personality? Are we possibly overfeeding some parts of the brain while keeping other parts undernourished?

"Our brain: an intricate, calibrated system of electrochemical signals, the incredible magic of ultimate design!"

Dr. Hans: Well, that's an interesting twist! Let's examine that from the scientific angle. Let's take a look at the ultimate computer, the human brain: three pounds of soft, pinkish gray tissue with 50 to 100 billion brain cells, something like a group of computers hooked together by complex circuits and feedback loops to hold all the memories, our understanding of the world, our dreams— an intricate, calibrated system of electrochemical signals, the incredible magic of ultimate design!

Brain anatomists have been able to map out the brain in great detail. They have discovered, for instance, that a rainbow is seen at the back of the brain, for that's where the screen is. And they found that a kiss is *felt* on the **sensory** strip.

LaVerne: So it really is all in the head after all?

Dr. Hans: O sure! It certainly is. This sensory strip is an arch across the cerebral cortex, the outer layer of the brain. It is here on the sensory strip that sensory information, signals from the skin, bones, joints, and muscles everywhere in the body, are received. Once they are received, they are interpreted in a fraction of a millisecond, and then processed by the **motor** strip, an arch of brain tissue situated parallel to the sensory strip. It is this motor strip where specific cell groups control specific muscle groups. For instance, moving your knee is initiated by cells close to the top of the motor strip, whereas moving your lips is initiated by cell groups in the lower portion.

And just note how much of each arch is devoted to each area of the body—the size of a section corresponds not to the size of the body part but to the precision with which it must be controlled for various tasks.

Look how much brain tissue the lips take up for sensory and especially for motor function in order to make possible the great precision that the lips require in word formation, in expressions, and, yes, even in how you kiss!

LaVerne: Absolutely amazing, isn't it? But tell me something about that frontal part of the brain, that white area. What happens here?

Dr. Hans: Let's go to Harvard University to find out what happens in the front brain, in the frontal lobes.

While Phineas Gage was tamping blasting powder with an iron rod, the dynamite exploded and shot the rod, like a long bullet, up just below his eye right through the front of his brain and out the top of his head! Surprisingly, his wound healed and he recovered. But Phineas was no longer Phineas!

According to his physician at Harvard, Phineas, while formerly known for his dependability and devotion to his family, now became irresponsible, irreverent, and a man of angry outbursts. In fact, he lost his job. He also lost his love for his family, leaving them to go to South America, where he existed in a whirl of wine, women, and song. The

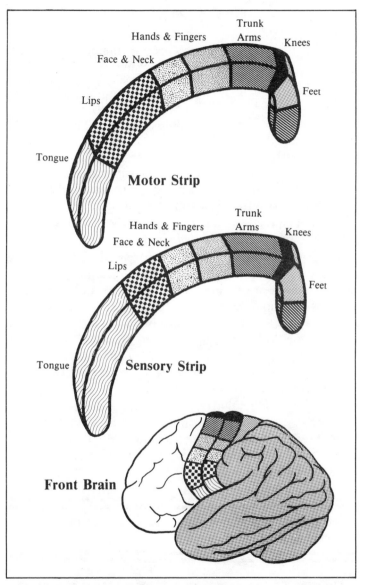

FIG. 2.1: The Brain, its Motor and Sensory Strips
Portions of these brain strips are devoted to different areas of the body. Strip portion does not correspond to the size of the body part but to the precision that's needed.

accident had actually changed his personality and even his character.

Although his intelligence skills and memory remained intact, his frontal lobes were ruined; and with that he lost his willpower, his values. *His moral and spiritual nature changed.* The taproot of his personality had been cut!

LaVerne: You are saying that the large frontal lobes of the brain are related to personality, judgment and character?

Dr. Hans: Exactly! Dr. Luria, a leading Russian brain scientist, called the frontal lobe "the superstructure above all parts of the brain performing a universal function of general regulation of behavior and self-control."

Dr. Bernell Baldwin, a brain physiologist, calls the frontal lobe "the front seat driver of the brain."

You see, the front brain is something like a symphonic conductor. The conductor makes the difference: instead of noise, we have music, instead of jealousy and hate we can have balance and order!

While the other portions of the brain are largely concerned with information gathering, processing and storing, *the front brain represents a balancing organ, a shaper and seat of personality, temperament and character, a spiritual filter,* if you please.

LaVerne: That reminds me of the studies done on soldiers with shrapnel wounds of the brain. In some 200 soldiers the front brain had been damaged, and with that came an impairment of the will, more self-centeredness and a change in their values.

"The front brain is the front seat driver of the brain, a spiritual filter."

Dr. Hans: What many people don't realize is that you don't have to impair your front brain by violent means. You can influence it by what you feed it. Some scientists are concerned that much of today's formal education is mostly occupied in providing facts and figures, and many times just a bunch of impractical trivia.

These scientists are afraid that it may be difficult to develop properly a balanced character and personality if we don't feed the front brain with the great principles of responsibility, self-control, love and nobility of purpose.

Could it be that some portions of our brain become overfed while our front brain is undernourished?

LaVerne: Friend, computer scientists have taught us a fascinating principle of cause and effect, and they put it quite neatly: GARBAGE IN — GARBAGE OUT!

Friend, what are you feeding the finest computer ever built, your mind? Are you feeding it

    —guns and murders
    —family violence
    —soap operas
    —allurements
    —alcohol?

Or are you feeding it

    —the Bread of Life
    —courage and integrity (from great inspirational
        biographies)
    —family togetherness
    —appreciation and gratitude (When did you last
        surprise your spouse with a bouquet of flowers?)
    —helping others?

Dr. Hans: The front brain was made for great principles, noble motives and unselfish service. Thinking, planning and working for others is part of its role.

We all need more faith, courage, love, enthusiasm. These principles can create enduring brain circuits that tie the whole brain together electronically into a fully functioning balanced computer network. By consistent wholesome living, by creative reflection, by worshiping a loving Creator-Master Designer, by helping others, you are really investing in the finest computer operation around—your very own front brain.

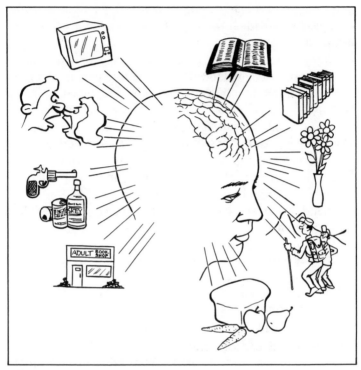

FIG. 2.2:
The Brain becomes what we feed it . . .

LaVerne: That is tremendous!

Friend, isn't it amazing to look at life through the discoveries of science, even at the front brain? And to realize again how wise the Good Book is when it emphatically emphasizes in Philippians 4:8: "Finally, whatever things are true, . . . honest, . . . pure, . . . lovely, . . . of good report, . . . *think on these things.*"

There is no higher, better, more interesting and truly enlightening way to build a well-balanced life than through the discovery of these lasting principles found through regular study of the Word of God. Introduce these divine principles to your children, because this way God builds mature and balanced men and women. Then discover for yourself the sweep and power, the depth and grandeur of this Book of books.

Friend, if you will approach this Book with a sincere and teachable spirit, you will be brought in touch with its Author, and there is no limit to the possibilities of your development!

In its wide range of style and subjects, the Bible has something to interest every mind and appeal to every heart. In its pages are found history, the most ancient; biography, the truest of life; principles of government for the control of the state, for the regulation of the household—principles that human wisdom has never equaled. It contains philosophy, the most profound, and poetry, the sweetest, the most sublime, the most impassioned.

The central theme of the Bible, the theme about all others in the whole book clusters, is the redemption plan, the restoration in the human soul of the image of God. The burden of every book and every passage of the Bible is the unfolding of this wondrous theme: how God loves and helps men and women to find a balanced and truly satisfying life.

Before you unfolds an infinite field for study. You have the key that will unlock to you the whole treasure house of God's Word.

You see, *the mind, the soul is built up by that upon which it feeds; and it rests with us to determine upon what it shall be fed.* It is within the power of everyone to choose the topics that shall occupy our thoughts and shape our characters.

With the Word of God in your hands, whatever your lot may be, you may have companionship as you choose. In its pages you may hold conversation with the noblest and best of the human race, and you may listen to the voice of the Eternal as He spoke to men and women. As you study and meditate upon the themes into which "the angels desire to look," you may have their companionship. You may follow the steps of the heavenly Teacher, and listen to His words when He taught on mountain and plain and sea. You may dwell in this world in the atmosphere of heaven, imparting to earth's sorrowing and tempted ones—members of

your family and loved ones, neighbors and friends—
thoughts of hope and longings for wholeness. And all the
time you yourself will be coming closer and still closer into
fellowship with the Unseen, all the time walking with God.
Make this your choice today.

*"Finally, whatever things are true, honest, pure, lovely, of
good report, think on these things." Philippians 4:8.*

3

Freedom Through Forgiveness

LaVerne: Dr. Hans, I know that you are quite concerned about the close relationship between the Western diet and the development of heart disease. It's a killer disease that is epidemic in our society, but very rare in those countries of the world where people practice a simpler dietary lifestyle and where they just live differently.

To me one of the most astounding facts about heart disease is that it evolves so gradually, so much so that many of us don't even know that we are building our case over time.

If I remember right, you said in one of your seminars that for many Americans the very first sign of heart disease is sudden death—they never had a symptom until the heart attack hit! It's really a disease, then, that creeps up on us in an insidious manner!

Dr. Hans: The tragedy is that with our rich diet we can build our case of progressive atherosclerosis, hardening of the arteries, by the forkfull. But since the evolving disease doesn't show up for decades, we don't often make the connection between diet and disease and so are stunned when the heart attack hits!

LaVerne: You mentioned that this hardening of the arteries usually leads to "arterial rust" and vessel blockage which then can interfere with proper blood flow, leading to disease and death. What about hardening of our attitudes and our emotions? Do they have an effect on our health?

Dr. Hans: O sure they do! Let me share with you a fascinating experiment by Dr. Harold Wolff that showed how emotions can influence our physical well-being.

Dr. Wolff, a well-known physician, had taken care of Tom. Tom had undergone some surgery to his stomach, but the incision to his stomach did not want to heal. This wound then allowed his physician to look into the inside of his stomach and to observe the digestion of different foodstuffs. And then it happened: by sheer accident, Dr. Wolff one day observed that the stomach lining was deep red instead of the usual pink color and was greatly engorged. At the same time he noticed that Tom was quite upset. Could the patient's emotional state have anything to do with his stomach changes?

Here is what Dr. Wolff found: Every time Tom was calm and relaxed, his stomach would look pink and appear calm and relaxed. But whenever Tom became angry and turned red, his stomach would also turn red, become engorged and secrete large amounts of gastric acid.

Since those early observations, we now know that some people can respond to harbored emotions with asthma, migraine headaches, ulcers, and even angina attacks.

Emotions then can break down the life force and invite disease and death! Or they can promote health, depending on the kind of emotion.

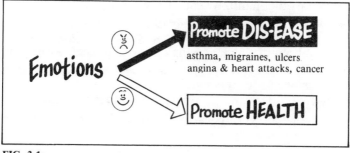

FIG. 3.1:
Effect of Emotion on Health and Disease

LaVerne: Our health and happiness then depend in part on how we react to life's challenges and how we solve daily problems!

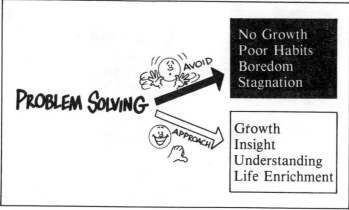

FIG. 3.2:
The Effect of Problem Solving on Life.

Dr. Hans: That's right. It's this whole process of solving problems that gives life meaning. *Through the often painful struggle of solving problems we grow mentally, emotionally, and spiritually and develop deeper insights.* Those things that hurt may instruct and teach us! Wise people, therefore, lear bravely, cheerfully to accept problems and even the pain of problems.

On the other hand, we can also still try to avoid problem-solving, sometimes even blaming others for our problems. Instead of dealing with problems, getting through them, we try to get out of them, rationalize them away, ignore, deny or drown them. But that diminishes us: we lose out on the richness of life, on personal growth, on inner healing, on shared victories, and in greater self-understanding.

LaVerne: Stress forces growth, and growth leads to insight and understanding.

Dr. Hans: Yes. We would remain spineless worms, like the caterpillar in the cocoon, if we didn't have to flex our muscles against the "walls" of difficulty and hardship in life.

I believe that what happens to us is not so important as how we perceive and relate to it! *Experience will make us either "bitter" or "better." Only one letter makes the difference, the letter "I," our ego.*

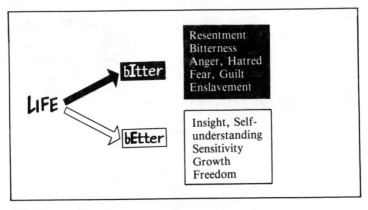

FIG. 3.3:
Coping with Life.

If we are mostly concerned about our *rights,* then the doors are wide open for resentment, bitterness, anger, hatred, fear, guilt. These are self-destructive emotions that are foremost in depleting our emotional energies. And these are the very blockages which stunt the life-giving streams of human interaction and cause our spirit to shrivel. You may call it "spiritual atherosclerosis,"—hardening of the spiritual arteries—hardening of the attitudes!

Let me give you an example of how these emotions can destroy us. A patient came to see me ostensibly about her depression and binge eating. However, only fifteen minutes into the interview she had to tell me all about her husband's affair with his nurse some thirteen years previously. She had become totally obsessed with the other woman. She had her tracked. She even knew her weight. She resented her for what she had done to her more than a decade ago. She hated her. Bitterness, hate, resentment—the instinctive means of revenge—created an emotional focus toward that person. It dominated her thoughts, emotions, and decisions, giving her severe depression.

LaVerne: But that didn't help to restore her marital relationship either, did it?

Dr. Hans: No. It distracted her from developing herself! It was the "poor me" story, feeling sorry for herself instead of processing the pain, finding a new level of balance and harmony in her life. And when she finally gained some insight, she summarized it well: "The moment I started to hate that woman, I became her slave. I couldn't enjoy my work anymore because she controlled my thoughts. I became fatigued. The work I once enjoyed became drudgery. Even vacations ceased to be a joy. I couldn't escape her tyrannical grasp on my mind until I focused on my life and what I was going to do with it."

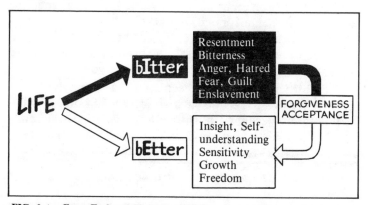

FIG. 3.4: **From Enslavedom to Freedom!**

LaVerne: What a tragic waste! What she needed was to turn her anger and bitterness into forgiveness, clear the record and find freedom and release.

Dr. Hans: However, that is the difficult part. Until we see that the offense may have actually been a benefit in disguise—forcing personal growth, insight, and sensitivity—we remain in our prisons of destructive emotions!

LaVerne: Which reminds me of the story of Mrs. Hannah. She resented the verdict of "lifetime in prison." Why could he live when her daughter had to be dead? She threw darts at his picture. She hated him more than she did anybody else. And yet she was totally unaware that she herself was becoming imprisoned in her own prison of hate.

But then one day the Gideon Bible Society, involved in prison ministry, asked her to address a Bible to the killer of her daughter. "I can't do it! I can't forgive him!" she blurted out. "But how can God forgive you if you cannot forgive others?" the Gideon asked with sincerity.

"Hardening of the attitudes, spiritual atherosclerosis, stunt the life-giving streams of human interaction."

Over the following weeks her conviction grew that the minister had been right at the gravesight service when he said, "It was meant for evil, but good may come from it!" When she prayed for forgiveness for her own feelings of hate, she finally found release! She even included with the Bible a note saying "Mrs. Hannah loves you."

The murderer had never been told that someone loved him—never ever! It made such an impression on him that he ultimately became a born-again Christian. He became a preacher to his fellow convicts. Love had changed his life.

"Hardening of our spiritual arteries causes our spirit to shrivel."

Now love could be shared with others. But the love note also changed Mrs. Hannah. The old embittered Mrs. Hannah died and a new Mrs. Hannah lived. Why? Because she discovered peace and freedom through forgiveness and acceptance.

"Problems and offenses may be benefits in disguise, forcing personal growth, insight and sensitivity, enriching life."

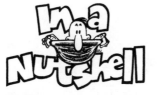

TO SUMMARIZE: Life is an endless series of problems. We can moan or we can solve them. We can resent or hate problems and thus deprive ourselves of personal growth and healing, or we can learn to face problems, experience pain, and learn from the experience. To learn we must:

1. *Accept responsibility.* Don't blame others. Process the problems in due time. The longer you ignore the problems, the larger they get.

2. *Dedicate yourself to truth.* Constant truthfulness gives freedom from fear and reduces confusion in the world. Truth means stringent self-examination, facing the consequences, with total honesty. Do not minimize.

3. *Talk to an understanding friend.*

4. *Ask for and offer forgiveness* even to the party that wronged you.

5. *Concentrate on positive emotions:* joy, peace, love, patience, gratitude.

6. *"Work" toward change.* Remember: healing often involves being willing to accept and process pain rather than to inflict pain.

So, friend, although the pain may be deep, invite Jesus into your life to remove the blockages that may have influenced your attitudes toward life and others, to remove resentment, hate, guilt, anger, bitterness, and to give you peace and freedom through His forgiveness. Welcome Him in! He can do it! He will do it!

4

Proven in Death

LaVerne: In my world travels I have learned that the incidence of diabetes is much lower in most countries than it is in the United States [our country]. And I was amazed to learn recently that blood sugar levels of diabetics can be normalized. As a matter of fact, I have been told that most diabetics who develop the disease in adulthood could get off insulin if only they would eat a more natural plant food diet and get into a regular daily walking program!

Dr. Hans: You will be even more amazed when you learn that as far back as 1930, Dr. Rabinowitch from Montreal demonstrated in hundreds of patients that a low fat, basically vegetarian diet could normalize diabetes in weeks.

Unfortunately, this simple and effective treatment never became the standard treatment for diabetes because it was overshadowed by the discovery of insulin, which appeared at the time to be the ultimate and heroic answer! It took until 1970 for Nathan Pritikin to rediscover the work of Dr. Rabinowitch and to propagate it as a simple and effective treatment method.

LaVerne: Now, if I understand this correctly, Pritikin claimed that some changes in our diet and exercise patterns could minimize the risk and severity of diabetes, heart disease and obesity. Right?

Dr. Hans: That's correct. Nathan Pritikin believed and asserted with great vigor that these western chronic diseases were due largely to our rich diet, a diet high in fats and oils, in animal products and in salt and sugar.

But he went further: on the basis of hundreds of animal experiments and many observations in different human populations in the world as well as on his own experiments, he announced to the world in 1976 that heart disease was reversible.

Almost thirty years ago Nathan Pritikin lived the great American dietary lifestyle: he enjoyed the ice creams, the french fries, the eggs, the steaks—and he paid a very dear price for it. When he was forty-two years of age he was diagnosed as having not only lymphatic cancer, apparently due to x-ray treatments he received for some skin condition, but also severe coronary artery disease due to atherosclerosis, a condition which prevents sufficient blood from reaching the heart.

When Nathan Pritikin asked his cardiologist whether he could do something to lower his high cholesterol levels, he was advised that cholesterol levels could not be changed. "Whay you have, you have." When he asked about exercise, he was told to walk no more than fifty yards at a time. "It will kill you if you do. Take it easy!" But take it easy was one thing Nathan Pritikin could not do. Determined to find answers, he began his own dietary experiments on his own body. To his astonishment, he found that his cholesterol level, far from being fixed, had actually dropped thirty to forty per cent as a result of his change in diet. He also discovered that as he began to exercise, carefully at first, he didn't drop dead but became stronger every day. He was actually eating himself and walking himself into better health.

Nathan Pritikin

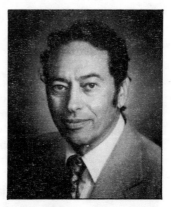

It was his personal improvement and the results of his Long Beach study of a group of heart disease patients who followed his diet that emboldened him in 1976 to announce to the world that he had reversed heart disease.

He tried to show angiographic documentation, but he was laughed at. The scientific and medical communities looked skeptically at this man, keenly aware that he had no medical and educational credentials, only a searching mind. Everyone "knew" that atherosclerosis—hardening of the arteries—was an irreversible process.

When he made his pronouncements about the reversibility of heart disease, he became at once a marked man: government agencies and medical organizations looked at him as an outsider, a "crusader." To them, Nathan Pritikin, was indeed a controversial man. But despite professional skepticism he continued to advance his ideas and started his rehabilitation program whereby he demonstrated in pioneering experiments the efficacy of his approach.

In addition, he wrote four major books that became best sellers, exhorting Americans to simplify their lifestyle and then to avoid typically Western diseases, such as high blood pressure, diabetes, heart disease, cancer and gallstones, and urging them instead to eat a simpler diet and to live with all their heart!

It was the success of this approach that became later reflected in the *U. S. Dietary Goals* recommending that

Americans change their diet: double the intake of starchy foods like grains and potatoes and eat less animal products, sugar, salt and fats.

LaVerne: It was because of the emerging recognition of his work that a real shock came not too long ago when Nathan Pritikin at the age of 69 committed suicide. Thousands of Americans were shaken at the news that the man who had helped many others couldn't save himself and so died at his own hand when he learned he had terminal leukemia. What actually happened?

Dr. Hans: When his leukemia surfaced again, he underwent a careful clinical evaluation at a university medical center. He was advised that the best treatment available was Interferon, a very powerful, very expensive, yet promising drug. He took it, and the results were most tragic.

Within ten weeks his health was deeply impaired, the medication ultimately leading to liver and kidney failure. Dialysis and other last-minute interventions took place; but it was too late. The life of a lifesaver was ebbing away. At the end, Nathan Pritikin, who had taken charge of his disease so valiantly, now took charge of his own death. Senator McGovern in the eulogy called him a "bold pioneer, perhaps the greatest lifesaver that lived in the 20th century." He said that there was no man so disciplined in the service of others.

"Nathan Pritikin was a man of great dedication, unusual humility, a bold pioneer, perhaps the greatest lifesaver that lived in the 20th century." —Senator George McGovern

---

The *New England Journal of Medicine* gave the autopsy report a few weeks later. The pathologist at the New York hospital who performed the autopsy was absolutely thunderstruck when he found the coronary arteries as clean as the arteries of a ten-year-old boy. In a man 69 years old who 27 years ago had been diagnosed as having a coronary artery disease, the near absence of atherosclerosis and the complete absence of its effects were a most remarkable finding!

Isn't it interesting that here was a man who had to prove in his own death that the common American disease called atherosclerosis is indeed reversible; that not only can you create your own disease, but you can reverse if it you are willing to follow a more simple dietary lifestyle!

LaVerne: You know, two thousand years ago a Man died on a cross. He, too, was considered controversial. He asserted that God was love, that He had come to vindicate God as a loving God, a good God, a God able and willing to give everything He had so that we can live.

He also brought into focus the *Good Book as the engineering manual for happiness and harmony.* And He went about healing those that were sick in body and soul.

He, too, was criticized. He, too, suffered from ecclesiastical jealousy of His day. He, too, was laughed at and suffered official skepticism. There was a public controversy and person rejection of Him. And we nailed Him to the cross. When He laid down His life willingly, the scoffers were there mocking Him: "He saved others; but He cannot save Himself." He died; He laid down His life for us that we might be clean. He removed the atherosclerosis of sin so that we can live clean lives. He opened up the channels of love. He taught us that our sins, though they are as scarlet, are forgiven and forgotten and we don't have to hang onto the guilt that is always with us. We are clean. We stand before God with clean hearts because we believe in the *ultimate Lifesaver and the ultimate Lifegiver*—Jesus Christ Himself.

Friend, I would like to recommend that ultimate Lifegiver and Lifesaver to you. He can make all the difference. Accept Him; He will not let you down!

Nathan Pritikin's Heart

Adapted from *The New England Journal of Medicine*
July 4, 1985

To the Editor: Nathan Pritikin and the principles he publicized have been of interest to physicians for some time. His work has been discussed in many forums, including the *Journal*. Mr. Pritikin died in February 1985 at the age of 69, and we wish to report the clinical and autopsy findings.

In February 1958, the diagnosis of coronary artery disease was made during a comprehensive medical evaluation. In a special cardiac assessment test, the electrocardiogram showed clear evidence of coronary artery disease. This diagnosis was confirmed by another test in December of 1959.

Mr. Pritikin's fasting blood cholesterol level was 280 mg% in December of 1955, and it was at that time that he started to experiment with different diets. At the time of diagnosis of coronary artery disease (1958), he formulated and began to follow the Pritikin high-complex carbohydrate, low fat, and low cholesterol diet. His blood cholesterol levels since 1955 are as follows:

Dec. 1955: 280 mg%	Feb. 1958: 210 mg%
July 1958: 162 mg%	June 1960: 120mg %
Dec. 1963: 102 mg%	Sept. 1968: 118 mg%
Jan. 1969: 112 mg%	Nov. 1984: 94 mg%

Mr. Pritikin led a vigorous life, and until late 1984 he ran several miles daily. In 1958, Mr. Pritikin had a malignant lymphoma. Intermittent chemotherapy provided control for several years. In 1984 and 1985 several experimental agents were tried, which caused several severe complications. Mr. Pritikin died in February of 1985.

An autopsy revealed lymphoma in partial remission and several findings caused by the drug treatment. The cardiovascular findings were as follows:

All coronary arteries were soft and pliable without any evidence of atherosclerotic plaques or a narrowing of these vessels. There was no evidence of any infarction.

All other major arteries were also soft and pliable without any evidence of atherosclerotic plaques or vessel narrowing.

There was no evidence of any vascular disease.

In a man 69 years old, the absence of developed atherosclerosis and the complete absence of its effects are remarkable.

Jeffrey D. Hubbard, M.D.
Bender Hygienic Laboratory

Stephen Inkíles, M. D., M.P.H.
Ocean View Medical Group

R. James Barnard, Ph.D.
Pritikin Research Foundation

Appendix

GOOD SOURCES OF SELECTED NUTRIENTS

NUTRIENT	GOOD SOURCES
Vitamin A	Dark-green and yellow vegetables; yellow fruit.
Vitamin C	Fruits, especially cantaloupe, lemons, grapefruit, oranges, tangerines, strawberries; raw cabbage, sweet peppers, tomatoes, potatoes.
Vitamin D	Direct sunshine; fortified milk.
Niacin	Whole-grain and enriched breads and cereals; legumes; potatoes; green vegetables.
Riboflavin	Green, leafy vegetables; whole-grain products; prunes; milk.
Thiamin	Whole-grain products; peas; beans; wheat germ; potatoes; leafy vegetables; brewer's yeast.
Iron	Legumes; whole-grain cereal and breads; dried fruits; green leafy vegetables.
Calcium and Phosphorus	Greens: mustard, kale, turnip tops, cabbage, broccoli; whole-grain products; citrus fruits; skimmed milk products.

Common Measurement Equivalents

1 tablespoon	= 3 teaspoons
1/8 cup (1 fluid ounce)	= 2 tablespoons
¼ cup	= 4 tablespoons
⅓ cup	= 5⅓ tablespoons
½ cup	= 8 tablespoons
⅔ cup	= 10⅔ tablespoons
¾ cup	= 12 tablespoons
1 cup (8 fluid ounces)	= 16 tablespoons
1 pint	= 2 cups
1 quart	= 2 pints (4 cups)
1 gallon	= 4 quarts
1 pound	= 16 ounces

CHOLESTEROL CONTROL

Cholesterol Content of Selected Food Items

Cholesterol is found only in foods of animal origin, such as meat, fish, poultry, eggs, and dairy items. The highest concentration exists in internal organs, egg yolk and shellfish. Plant products do not contain any cholesterol. The amount of cholesterol in breads, desserts, and combination foods depends upon the amount of milk, eggs and dairy products used in the recipe. In addition to containing cholesterol, foods of animal origin are also frequently high in saturated fats, which raise the body's cholesterol production by the liver.

It is recommended that you choose a diet low in total fat. Saturated fat, especially, should be avoided. Cholesterol intake recommendations should be consistent with the level of serum cholesterol levels in your blood. As a general guideline, serum cholesterol levels should ideally be 100 mg% plus age. An ideal serum cholesterol level for a man 55 years of age therefore would be 100 plus 55 = 155 mg%. To accomplish these ideal levels of serum cholesterol, it is important to keep the dietary cholesterol intake ideally below 100 mg/day. The list below will provide you with some figures of which foods you should use only sparingly. Try to emphasize vegetables, fruits, whole grains, legumes and skimmed milk products in your diet. If you are used to meat in your diet, then try to reduce to the point that you use it more as a condiment and as a flavoring agent rather than the mainstay of the meal. Low fat meats, of course, are preferable.

Cholesterol Content of Selected Foods (in mg)

MEAT AND POULTRY:

Beef, pork, chicken	5 oz.	135
Liver	3 oz.	370
Sweetbreads	3 oz.	400
Frankfurter	3 oz.	50
Bologna	3 oz.	85
Liverwurst	3 oz.	105

FISH AND SEAFOOD:

Crabs, Lobsters, Shrimp	1 cup	120
Halibut, Salmon, Tuna	5 oz.	80
Sardines	5 oz.	80

EGGS:

Egg Yolk	1	250
Egg White	1	0

DAIRY PRODUCTS:

Skim Milk, Buttermilk	1 cup	5
Whole Milk	1 cup	34
Ice cream	1 cup	110
Cottage Cheese, creamed	1 cup	50
uncreamed	1 cup	15

DESSERTS:

Custard, baked	1 cup	280
Cream Puffs	1	190
Sponge Cake	1 sl.	165
Lemon Meringue pie	1 sl.	100

FATS, OILS, SPREADS:

Bacon, Canadian	4 sl.	80
Butter	1 Tbsp.	35
Mayonnaise	1 Tbsp.	10

FAT CONTROL

Fat Content of Selected Food Items (in mg)

FOOD	(% Fat of Calories)	FOOD	(% Fat of Calories)
Milk: Skim	2	Vegetables	1-5
Whole	50	Fruits	1-5
Ice Cream	55	Tubers	1-10
Cheeses: Cottage	36	Legumes	5-10
Past. Processed	60-85	Grains	5-15
Cream Cheese	90	Soy: Beans	40
Chicken, Turkey	15-40	Tofu	50
Fish	15-40	Meat Analogs	50-80
Beef, Pork	65-83	Choc. Candy	50-60
Bacon	85-94	Nuts	75-90
		Olives, Avocados	90

Hidden Fats

FOOD (Producer)	Total Calories	Fat Calories	% Fat of Cals.
Hungry Man Veal. Parm. (Swanson, 20 oz.)	700	306	43
Hungry Man Turkey Pie (Swanson, 16 oz.)	800	423	53
Steak House Frozen Beef (Morton)	890	576	65
T-Bone Platter (Rustler)	952	477	50
T-Bone Steak (untrimmed, 8 oz.)	1072	890	83
Triple Cheeseburger (Wendy's, 14 oz.)	1080	620	60

Fat Content of Some Low Fat Cheeses

Cheese	Amount	Calories	Gms. of Fat
Borden's Lite-Line	1 oz.	50	2.0
Chef's Delight	1 oz.	70	4.0
Cottage Cheese, dry curd	4 Tbsp.	56	0.2
Countdown	1 oz.	40	1.0
Hoop Cheese	½ cup	80	1.0
Kraft Light n' Lively	1 oz.	70	4.0
Ricotta	1 oz.	45	3.0
Sapsago	1 oz.	30	.4
Weight Watcher's Cheese	1 oz.	50	2.0

SUGAR CONTROL

- Hide the sugar bowl
- Save candy, cake, pies and cookies for special occasions
- Eat "crunchy munchies" of fruits and vegetables
- Read the labels; where is sugar in the list?
- Buy canned fruits in own or light juice instead of heavy syrup. Better yet, use fresh fruit!

Sugar Content of Selected Food Items

Food	Size Portion	Teaspoons of Sugar
BEVERAGES		
Soda Pop, Cola drinks		
Ginger Ale, Sweet Cider	12 oz.	8-11
JAMS AND JELLIES		
Jelly	2 Tbsp.	10
Marmalade, jams	2 Tbsp.	10
CANDIES		
Marshmallow	10	15
Hard candy	4 oz.	20
Chocolate milk bar	3 oz.	5
Chocolate mints	4	8
Fudge	2 oz. sq.	9
FRUIT AND CANNED JUICES		
Raisins	½ cup	4
Fruit Cocktail (commercial)	1 cup	10
Orange Juice (unsweetened)	1 cup	4
Grape Juice (commercial)	1 cup	7
BREADS, CAKES, COOKIES		
Hamburger Bun, Hot Dog Bun	1	3
German Chocolate Cake	1 (8 oz.)	15
Angel, Pound Cake	1 (6 oz.)	9
Chocolate cookies	4	6
Ginger Snaps	4	12
Chocolate eclair	1	7
Donut (glazed)	1	6
DAIRY PRODUCTS		
Ice Cream, Sherbet	1 cup	6-8
Ice Cream Cone, empty	1 triple	10
Chocolate milk	1 cup	8
PIES & PUDDINGS		
Jello	1 cup	9
Pies: Apple, Berry, Cherry, Coconut,		
Custard	1 slice	10
Raisin	1 slice	13
Puddings: Chocolate, Rice	1 cup	8-10

SODIUM CONTROL

Sodium Content of Selected Foods

Food	Size Portion	Sodium (mg)
Milk	1 cup	120
Buttermilk	1 cup	280
Pasteurized Cheeses	2 slices	400
Cottage Cheese	½ cup	470
Roquefort	¼ cup	470
Pimiento Cheese Spread	1 oz.	470
Ham	1 oz.	265
Luncheon Meats	1 oz.	300
Veg. Luncheon "Meats"	1 oz.	375
Frankfurter	1	500
Bacon	3 slices	630
Melba Toast	6	225
RyKrisp	3	225
Cornbread	1½″ x 1½″	250
Cheerios	1 cup	250
All-Bran Cereal	1 cup	575
Waffles/Pancakes	2	400
Potato Chips	15—2″	300
Tomato Juice	1 cup	500
Ketch-up	3 Tbsp.	565
V-8 Juice	1 cup	825
Tomato Sauce	½ cup	830
Olives, green	6	575
Pepper Lemon (Durkee's)	1 tsp.	700
Salt	1 tsp.	2200

(The Daily Sodium Intake should not exceed 2000 mg = 5000 mg of Salt)

Sodium Content of Some Fast Foods

FAST FOOD	AVERAGE SODIUM CONTENT (mgs. per portion)
Hamburgers	
Burger King Whopper	990
Jack-in-the-Box Jumbo	1010
McDonald's Big Mac	960
Beef Sandwiches	
Arby's Roast Beef	870
Burger King Chopped Steak	965
Roy Rogers Roast Beef	610
Fish	
Arthur Treacher's	420
Burger King	970
Long John Silver	1335
McDonald's	710
Chicken	
Kentucky Fried 3-piece Dinner	2285
Other Specialty Items	
Jack-in-the-Box Taco Meal	925
Pizza Hut Pizza Supreme	1280
Wendy's Chili	1190

HOW TO CUT THE SALT AND NOT THE TASTE

Unsalted foods can be made more tasty if skillful use of herbs and spices is practiced. Here are some suggestions:

1. In experimenting with herbs, use no more than ¼ teaspoon of dried herbs, or ¾ teaspoon of fresh herbs for a dish that serves four people.

2. To soups and stews that are cooked a long time (crockpots), add herbs during the last hour of cooking.

3. When cooking vegetables or making sauces and gravies, cook herbs along with them.

4. To cold foods such as tomato juice, salad dressings, and cottage cheese, add herbs several hours before serving. You may store these foods in the refrigerator for 3 to 4 hours or overnight.

5. Remember—The correct combinations of herbs and spices for any food is the one that tastes best to you.

Let me emphasize again—don't over season, as vegetables have wonderful flavors in their own right.

A very versatile seasoning is "Mrs. Dash." Use the one without salt, and low pepper.

VEGETABLE SEASONING SUGGESTIONS

Asparagus—lemon juice, chives, thyme, tarragon

Beans, dried—bay leaf, garlic, marjoram, onion, oregano, thyme

Beans, green—basil, dill seed, thyme, onion, tarragon

Beets—lemon or orange juice or peel; ginger

Broccoli—lemon juice, dill, oregano

Cabbage—creole cabbage with tomatoes, green pepper, garlic and onion

Carrots—parsley, mint, dillweed, orange or lemon peel, poppy or sesame seed

Cauliflower—Italian seasonings, paprika, sesame or dill seed

Celery—stirfry with mild soy sauce, sesame seeds and tomato

Corn—bell pepper, pimiento, tomatoes, chives

Okra—try broiling for a crisp texture

Peas—mint, fresh mushrooms, pearl onions, sliced water chestnuts

Potatoes—parsley, chopped green pepper, onion, chives, dill

Spinach—lemon juice, mild vinegar, rosemary

Squash—bake with chopped apple and lemon juice

Tomatoes—sprinkle curry powder or parmesan cheese; broil with mushrooms, green pepper and onion

FURTHER RECOMMENDED READING

For more recipes we recommend:

Brody, Jane. *Jane Brody's Good Food Book: Living the High Carbohydrate Way.* NY: W. W. Norton, 1984. 702 p.

[1] Calkins, Fern. *It's Your World Vegetarian Cookbook.* Washington, D.C. Review & Herald Publishing Assoc., 1981. 304 p.

[2] Connor, Sonja & W. Connor. *The New American Diet.* New York: Simon & Schuster, 1986. 410 p.

[3] Cottrell, Edyth. *Oats, Peas, Beans & Barley Cookbook.* Santa Barbara: Woodbridge Press, 1981. 268 p.

[4] Dameron, Peggy. *The Joy of Cooking Naturally,* 11538 Anderson, Loma Linda, CA 92354, 1983. 150 p.

[5] Leonard, J. and E. Taylor *The Live Longer Cookbook:* NY: Grosset & Dunlap, 1977. 249 p.

[6] McDougall, John & M. McDougall. *The McDougall Plan for Super Health and Life-long Weight Loss.* Piscataway, NJ: New Century Publ., 1983. 340 p.

[7] Pritikin, N. and P. McGrady. *The Pritikin Program for Diet and Exercise.* New York: Grossett & Dunlap, 1979. 433 p.

Rachor, J. *Of These Ye May Freely Eat—a Vegetarian Cookbook.* Sunfield, MI: Family Health Publ., 1986. 91 p.

Robertson, L. et al. *Laurel's Kitchen.* Berkeley: Nigri Press, 1976. 508 p.

Total Health Foundation. *Total Health Cookery.* P. O. Box 5, Yakima, WA 98907, 1980. 221 p.

Thrash, Agatha. *Eat for Strength.* Harrisburg, PA: ACM (1-800-233-4450), 1979. 222 p.

Weimar Institute. *From the Weimar Kitchen.* P. O. Box A, Weimar, CA 95736, 1978. 120 p.

For more in-depth study:

Bailie, Ira. *An Ounce of Prevention.* Turlock, CA: Golden Valley Health Promotion Press. 1986, 225 p.

Bennett, Cleaves. *Control Your Blood Pressure Without Drugs.* NY: Doubleday. 1984, 395 p.

Subscripts 1-7 indicate contributors to the recipe section. Recipes adapted from these original sources are marked 1-7. See also p. 131.

Burkitt, Denis. *Eat Right to Stay Healthy.* NY: Arco Publishing, Inc. 1979, 126 p.

Califano, Joseph. *America's Health Care Revolution.* NY: Random House. 1986, 241 p.

Farquhar, John. *The American Way of Life Need Not Be Hazardous to Your Health.* NY: Norton & Co. 1978, 196 p.

Hausman, Patricia. *Jack Sprat's Legacy: The Science and Politics of Fat and Cholesterol.* NY: Richard Marek Publishers. 1981, 287 p.

Hur, Robin. *Food Reform: Our Desperate Need.* Austin: Heidelberg Publishers. 1975, 260 p.

Leonard, Jon et al. *Live Longer Now.* NY: Grosset & Dunlap. 1974, 196 p.

Trowell, Hugh C. and Denis P. Burkitt. *Western Diseases: Their Emergence and Prevention.* Cambridge, Mass.: Harvard University Press. 1981, 480 p.

White, Ellen G. *Health and Happiness.* The Quiet Hour, Redlands, CA 92373. 1982, 384 p.

Index

25 commercial stations, hundreds of repeater and cable stations, and by satellite in North America and the Philippines.

The format is a series of Bible studies with neighbors that covers the entire Everlasting Gospel. Other programs with specialists in the fields of nutrition and health, marriage, parenting, prophecy, and the sanctuary, blended together with the Tucker Family Singers, make a visit at the Tucker home (via television) each week a most pleasing and inspirational time.

Telling the Good News . . .
Through MISSION PROJECTS

To the millions of Asia, The Quiet Hour means funds for evangelistic meetings. Through these Quiet Hour sponsored meetings more than 20,000 souls annually have come to a knowledge of Jesus Christ, been baptized and united with God's remnant church.

To thousands in Borneo, Thailand, the Philippines, India, and South America, The Quiet Hour means churches, Jungle Chapels, and Lambshelters. More than 1,000 of these have been constructed and thousands more are needed. Each chapel now costs $2,000 and Lambshelters cost $1,000.

Telling the GOOD NEWS . . .
Through LITERATURE

For 100,000 homes in all parts of the world, The Quiet Hour means the monthly issue of *The Quiet Hour Echoes*—our radio and television magazine. To millions of readers, our little missionary booklets—43 in our Tiny Giant series and 41 in our Search series—are The Quiet Hour.

But The Quiet Hour radio, television, literature, and mission outreach could not be realized if it were not for the scores of dedicated volunteer workers, the 32 employees, the thousands of sacrificing boosters and prayer partners. And in the final analysis, it is God's blessing, His Spirit, working in and through each one that has made and will continue to make The Quiet Hour ministry effectual for the winning of souls in time's last hour.

Would You Like to Be a Partner?

Help spread the saving message of Christ to the millions. With your partnership—your prayers and generosity—and with the blessing of God, many more will have the opportunity to hear and know and be ready for Christ's glorious return.

You can help in The Quiet Hour's outreach by being a partner in reaching unreached people.

• Pray daily for *The Quiet Hour* radio, television, literature, and worldwide mission endeavors.

• Help make it possible for every person in North America to hear the weekly broadcast of The Quiet Hour.

• SEARCH television programs reach a potential audience of more than 20 million. Let's triple that audience for Christ.

• Fifty-four mission airplanes have been provided by our wonderful boosters. Because of recessions and insufficient funding, a number of planes have had to be dropped from mission service. Now we are endeavoring to help supply the means to operate ten aircraft to speed the message and the messenger to isolated areas in mission lands.

• Thousands of children and youth are longing for an education in one of our Christian schools in developing countries. Would you like to sponsor a child through the elementary, high school, or college grades?

• Providing funds for an evangelistic crusade in India or the Philippines has brought untold joy to thousands of Quiet Hour boosters and has brought more than 20,000 souls into the kingdom of God annually during the past five years. Hundreds of millions of precious souls need to be reached now before it is too late.

It's wonderful to be a partner with Christ in working for the salvation of souls and the hastening of His coming. In these last days it is time for us to redouble our consecration, our efforts, and our sacrifice.

As a Partner Your Prayers and Support
Are Deeply Appreciated.

THE QUIET HOUR
630 Brookside, Redlands, California 92373-4699

A Better

Way of Life

Is Waiting for you!

- **How can I live a happier and healthier life?**
- **What is going to happen in the future?**
- **How can I know that there is a God?**

You will receive absolutely free 24 *Way of Life* Bible lessons, and upon completion of the course a beautiful certificate.

The Bible Course that Answers your Questions

- - - - - - - - - - - - - - - - - -

☐ *Yes,* I want a better *Way of Life*. Please send the Bible lessons. I understand there is no cost or obligation.

Name _____

Address _____

City/State_____ ZIP _____

THE QUIET HOUR
630 Brookside, Redlands, CA 92373-4699

ABOUT THE QUIET HOUR

Telling the Good News . . .
Through RADIO

The Quiet Hour radio, television, literature, and worldwide mission outreach had its beginning in Portland, Oregon. Pastor J. L. Tucker made his first radio broadcast on July 7, 1937, over radio station KEX. Evidence of God's rich blessings was immediate. The thrice weekly broadcast quickly grew into a twice daily minsitry.

In 1943 The Quiet Hour moved to the Bay Area—first Berkeley and then Oakland, California. It was here in 1949 that The Quiet Hour pioneered in the field of television on KGO-TV with a prime time weekly telecast on Saturday nights. And it was all *live*—nothing recorded. What a challenge!

Berrien Springs, Michigan, became the headquarters of The Quiet Hour in 1954. Here the broadcast began to take wings to all parts of the country, and was officially organized as a nonprofit religious corporation, making it possible for The Quiet Hour to legally receive wills, legacies, and enter into trust agreements for the advancement of the gospel.

In September of 1959 The Quiet Hour moved its headquarters to Redlands, California. Again there was evidence of divine guidance as the self-supporting ministry expanded rapidly until today the broadcast is now released on more than 300 stations in North and Central America, Southern Asia, and the Philippines.

Telling the Good News . . .
Through TELEVISION

Though The Quiet Hour pioneered in the field of television ministry in 1949 and 1950, the Search telecast, produced by The Quiet Hour, was born in 1970. The half-hour telecast, with LaVerne and Alma Tucker as hosts, is now released on more than

CASSETTE TAPES

Tens of thousands have benefited from Dr. Diehl's seminars by becoming motivated to simplify their dietary lifestyle and to get into a daily exercise routine. The Quiet Hour is pleased to make available to you one of Dr. Diehl's high quality *Lifesaver* albums.

HOW TO STAY YOUNGER LONGER

Experience Dr. Diehl in this dynamic 8-hour seminar at a national convention. It will show you how to live with **all** your heart and free from debilitating diseases. An excellent gift item!

Full color album with 8 tapes, $54.95 (donation).

VIDEO CASSETTES

Experience Dr. Diehl in our four-part television series

TO YOUR HEALTH,

which has been our most popular program to date. This is the perfect gift for those who want to be inspired and motivated to live healthier lives.

Order this exciting series on video cassette. Specify VHS or BETA, $30.00 (donation price).

THE QUIET HOUR
630 Brookside Avenue,
Redlands, California 92373-4699

SEMINARS

Dr. Diehl welcomes the opportunity to reinforce the information in this book with his personal motivating presentations and seminars.

For scheduling information:
Audiences of corporations, associations, health professionals, educational institutions, churches, hopsitals, and all interested private groups are invited to contact:

Health Spectrum Seminars
P. O. Box 356
Millbrae, CA 94030
(415) 692-5167

ABOUT THE AUTHOR

Dr. Hans Diehl

As a National Institutes of Health supported research fellow in cardiovascular epidemiology at Loma Linda University, Dr. Diehl evaluated the impact of the Pritikin Longevity Center, where he had directed the Research and Health Education program.

As a post-doctoral scholar at the School of Public Health at the University of California at Los Angeles he contributed to the establishment of the UCLA Center for Health Enhancement. He holds a doctorate in Health Science with emphasis on Lifestyle Medicine and has a master's degree in Public Health Nutrition from Loma Linda University.

He has demonstrated and published results showing that most hypertensives, diabetics and heart disease patients can normalize their disease and become drug free within weeks by simplifying their customary lethal American diet. And that people can eat more and weigh less.

Dr. Diehl is much in demand as a stimulating, dynamic and entertaining communicator. As director and founder of the *Lifestyle Medicine Institute,* he is equally comfortable in addressing a national medical convention in Germany or the National Auto Dealers' Association Convention in San Francisco on how to increase profits through wellness strategies.

His aim is to demystify American medicine and to help people become winners at lifestyling—to live fuller, happier lives and to die later feeling younger.

He and his wife, Dr. Lily Diehl, and their children Byron and Carmen live in Loma Linda, California.

MAIL TODAY

Dear Dr. Diehl, I enjoyed your book. The three most helpful chapters were:
(please circle)

I: 1 2 3 4 5 6 7 8 9 **II:** 1 2 3 **III:** 1 2 3 4
Part IV: Appendix/Bibliography

As a result of reading your book/seeing your video films/listening to your seminar on tape/attending your seminar, I have made a commitment to make the following changes in my lifestyle:

_____

_____

_____

☐ Please send me a FREE copy of your **Lifeline** health letter.

☐ Please enroll me in the *Way of Life* lessons.

Name _____

Address _____

City _____ State _____ ZIP _____

Name _____

Address _____

The Quiet Hour
630 Brookside Avenue
Redlands, CA 92373-4699

Attn: Dr. Hans Diehl